The Ordinary Person's Guide to
Extraordinary
HEALTH
Jillie Collings

AURUM PRESS

For my lovely husband Bee, who has often kept me in bread and feathers during my research of health and other frontiers

First published 1993 by Aurum Press Ltd
10 Museum Street, London WC1A 1JS
Copyright © 1993 by Jillie Collings

A catalogue record for this book is available from the British Library

ISBN 1 85410 243 5

1   3   5   7   9   10   8   6   4   2
1993   1995   1997   1996   1994

Line drawings by Willow

Designed by Don Macpherson
Printed and bound in Great Britain by Hartnolls Ltd, Bodmin.

CONTENTS

FOREWORD

During my thirty years as a practitioner of alternative/complementary medicine, I have been interviewed many times for newspapers, television and radio. In the summer of 1984, when I embarked on writing my first series of books on health, I was interviewed by Jillie Collings. I was immediately impressed by the content of her questions and the obvious knowledge she had of complementary medicine. The interview was probably one of the most difficult I had ever had, as Jillie went into great depth with her questions and I had to be very accurate in the answers I gave.

At the end of the interview we had the opportunity to have an informal discussion and we found that we had a great mutual interest in the field of complementary medicine. I was so impressed with the interview and also with our talk afterwards that I asked Jillie if we could meet again for further discussion, and I was pleased we did, as I learned a great deal from her about various subjects within the wide field of complementary medicine.

I was very happy to have been asked to write a foreword for this excellent book. Jillie, who is a very well known writer on the subject of health, has drawn on her wide knowledge to show the reader how to live a healthy life. She also points out the responsibility each of us has to increase our own health, energy and happiness. Not only is this book very well written but it provides tremendous advice for good health in day-to-day living, and deals with difficult and sometimes confusing material in a way that is clear and easy to understand.

As a health writer myself and having read this book intently, I can only emphasize that *The Ordinary Person's Guide to Extraordinary Health* is essential reading for maintaining optimum health. As with many other books, dietary management is involved, but the reader will find that Jillie's views are realistic and practical, and that the advice given is justified by proven facts.

Today, all over the world, there is a great increase in the interest in alternative and complementary medicine, and the need for books such as this is much larger than one might think. With the enormous attacks on the three forms of energy that man lives by – Food, Water and Air – there are many challenges to overcome, and there is a hunger for advice on what the individual can do to maintain good health. If one can keep these three simple factors of health in order – and I only have to look at my mentors who have, and who have all reached a very old age – then it is worthwhile to take up the challenge. Over my thirty years in practice I have been advising just that, and time and time again I have seen the great rewards of investing in one's health.

Conventional medicine and alternative medicine have to go hand in hand; they both exist to relieve human suffering and it is extremely important that bridges are built between the two. It is encouraging that everywhere in the world the urge to do this is growing stronger. The aim of alternative/complementary medicine is to treat the body as a whole, mind, body and spirit. Jillie has tremendous insight into this and is really quite far ahead in her ideas, as she has devoted many, many years to studying how this can work for everyone. The advice in this excellent book will assist even doctors and practitioners in their work-loads. Their lives will be made a great deal easier when this book is read and its message understood.

I have mentioned many times in my work the balance of 'Yin and Yang', so well recognised by the Chinese. Yin is female, Yang is male. The latter I can see as orthodox medicine, often a little harsh, very intellectual and rather sophisticated. Alternative medicine is gentle, very intuitive and friendly – the Yin. The time has come for these two to be married, and it will be a very happy marriage because the purpose is not only to help human suffering, but also to help people understand how wonderful these bodies of ours are and what they will do for us if we look after them the very best we can.

I am very happy to be given the opportunity to be a little part of this book, as I myself have found help in the information and advice that Jillie is giving so freely to us all.

I hope it is widely read, as it will be a great blessing on the marriage of orthodox and alternative medicine.

Jan de Vries
'Auchenkyle'
Southwoods Road
Troon
Ayrshire
Scotland

1
*

YOU AND THE CURRENT HEALTH CRISIS

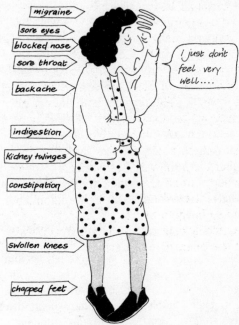

A BEWILDERING NUMBER OF PEOPLE SUFFER FROM MINOR AILMENTS.....

IN THIS CHAPTER

✳ Minor ailments – major signposts?   ✳ The challenge of
contemporary medicine   ✳ The changeover (from treating your
disease to treating you!)   ✳ The remarkable Robert Kowalski:
how he conquered his cholesterol problem   ✳ Helping yourself
to better health by moving the right molehill
✳ Your key role in the new health equation

A bewildering number of people today are suffering from a variety of symptoms and conditions for which regular medical treatment seems to have few, if any, answers. Yet when alternative medicine is tried, and more and more people are trying it, it doesn't always fill the breach.

Often the conditions and symptoms that cause people to seek treatment in the first place defy diagnosis. Tests are done and doctors reassure that there is no physical disease, but still there is discomfort, and often pain.

The symptoms persist, and they are not always relieved by medication. In fact, whenever medication is given the 'cure' is frequently worse than the condition: the drugs themselves have side effects, taking the edge off day-to-day life by inducing yet more symptoms such as drowsiness or indigestion. The phrase 'I just don't feel well' applies more and more to today's illnesses.

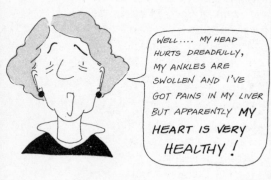

WELL.... MY HEAD HURTS DREADFULLY, MY ANKLES ARE SWOLLEN AND I'VE GOT PAINS IN MY LIVER BUT APPARENTLY MY HEART IS VERY HEALTHY !

What is happening? Should we ignore these so-called minor ailments? The ever-increasing incidence of visits to doctors' surgeries indicate that people don't think so. They sense, quite rightly, that if minor ailments are not addressed they can become major problems, and statistics certainly support this view. It is quite staggering, considering the extent and cost of modern healthcare and research, that by the year 2000 it has been estimated that one in three people will get cancer or heart/arterial disease. That's at least one person in every family. Yet coronary heart disease, one of the greatest killers in the West, was virtually unheard of at the turn of this century.

Clearly, our contemporary medical system is failing us, and what a blessing it is that there is now a revolution going on in the health world that will ultimately transform our understanding of illness and wellness and enable us to introduce more effective health care.

However, revolutions, especially health revolutions, take time to filter through to local consulting rooms. In the meantime, who is to pass on this new knowledge which can and will transform the health and well-being of the average individual, and do so safely, moreover, with few or no side effects?

Surely this is why more health books are being written now than ever before. Health writers such as myself figure that 'while the grass grows, the cow dies', so we are trying to dispense the new knowledge to fill the information gap, and also to pass on the good news that anyone can be healthy (or healthier) today with a minimum of effort. We don't have to live with our minor complaints, and we can make huge health inroads into our major ones too.

THE NEW HEALTH MOVEMENT

What is this new health movement? Names such as complementary, holistic and alternative are being used to describe it, but, if anything, they are only adding to the confusion. What they are trying to describe is that the new health system will be based on a belief that each part of the body is interdependent: you cannot separate the liver from the lungs or the head from the heart and try to cure the bit that's gone wrong, as our current (orthodox) system has been trying to do. In the past, we have been practising **organ**-based medicine – i.e. treatment based on the organ that's sick, such as the heart in heart trouble – but in the future we will be practising **system**-based medicine, because it has been recognized that the sick organ is merely the weakest link in a body system that is malfunctioning. So when in times to come you are diagnosed as having heart trouble, the whole of your circulatory system (heart, lungs, blood vessels etc.) will be overhauled. Furthermore, your circulatory system will then be placed into perspective with the your **WHOLE** body and its state of health. This is why the terms wholistic and holistic have been used to describe the new health movement, because they mean whole.

The new health movement will differ from the orthodox one in one other major way: it will concern itself with the healthy and not just with the sick. It is interested in preventing illness, not just in curing it. In this respect it follows ancient medical customs such as were once practised in China, where doctors were paid only if the patient stayed healthy!

In many ways the new movement is really a return to old ways, to folk medicine, to simple remedies, to natural foods and prophylactics. In the old days people used plants as foods and medicines, sometimes complemented by a bit of healing in the form of massage or a bit of stimulation such as applying hot or cold compresses to the body.

But whereas our ancestors did things because they knew they worked, their methods were a bit 'hit and miss' because they didn't always know why they worked. Someone just boiled up a few herbs and hoped for the best. Now, most of the time we know why, and we have the modern technology to make safer, surer remedies, and to understand their workings in the body.

3

NEW FORMS OF TREATMENT

We also have new ways of giving the body subtle energy boosts that will encourage it to do its own work of healing, rather than resorting to drugs or chemotherapy, which are often the physical equivalent of using a sledgehammer to crack a nut. Some futuristic machines will actually realign body energy in much the same way as you might tune a car. Such methods are designed to work with the body, coaxing and cajoling rather than pushing and shoving. Of course, orthodox techniques such as surgery will sometimes be needed and will always save lives, although chemotherapy has saved fewer people than we are led to believe. These techniques may always be needed when disease has gone so far that drastic measures are called for. No one is denying the value of orthodox medicine. But it is a rescue system, and the new health beliefs contend that this is its major fault: it does not start soon enough – that is, with the minor symptoms or even before them.

Hence the new health regime is based on the maxim, 'an ounce of prevention is worth a pound of cure'. It is based on individuals taking responsibility for their own health and not entirely relying on the doctor to keep sickness at bay. In that respect it is a do-it-yourself system.

KNOWLEDGE: KEY TO HEALTH

As such, it must incorporate one other vital ingredient: knowledge. We are all going to have to learn a little bit about the workings of the body if we are to know how to prevent it from malfunctioning. If you want to become an electrician, you don't start by putting your hand in the fuse box: you start by learning how electricity works.

Funnily enough, this analogy is especially appropriate, because the body **is** an electrical system, but it is not the strength of the electricity we receive in our houses: it is millions and millions of times weaker and more subtle and is, therefore, very susceptible to other kinds of electricity – hence all the current research into the long-term effects of using VDUs, cooking with microwave ovens, etc.

However, the body is tough and resilient too, and with a minimum of help and protection it can survive all, or nearly all, that modern life can throw at it.

Quite simply the time has come for each one of us to know what that help and protection is and to take our health in our own hands. After all, that's where the buck stops. When you are finally very ill, it's not the doctor who suffers the symptoms. It's you.

So this book is based on body systems, how they work and how to keep them healthy, plus any new approaches there may be for improving the more common complaints for each system. There are also suggestions about lifestyles – suggestions that may help you to choose healthier ways of running that bit of your life which may be contributing to your current health problems. It is no good tackling a body-system problem unless you also tackle the lifestyle factors that may have contributed to it.

THE SMALL CHANGE/BIG BONUS THEORY

Most people get a feeling of doom when somebody suggests that they change their lifestyle in any way, thinking that it usually means giving up a favourite vice such as drinking, smoking or eating, or giving up something even more impossible such as going to work because it makes you tense and could be viewed as a long-term health hazard!

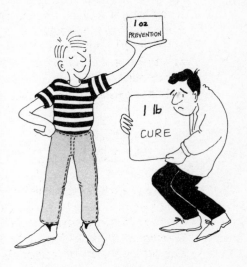

To make a change for the better in your health, it is often quite unnecessary to move mountains, just to move the right molehill. We have all seen those comedy sequences in which someone moves a linchpin and the whole caboodle changes shape. The body is so wonderful, so recuperative, that one small change can start a whole new trend in your life, which can then snowball, collecting debris from other seemingly insoluble life factors and sweeping them away as well.

Best-selling author Robert Kowalski, who wrote *The Eight Week Cholesterol Cure*, made just such a small change when, at 41, he had already had one major heart attack followed by two multiple by-pass operations, neither of which afforded him long-term improvement. He personally researched all the known remedies for his condition, however implausible they seemed. He completely cured his problem by taking a simple oat cereal everyday together with vitamin therapy (of which more in Chapters 4 and 7). Simple changes often work, while complex ones may produce their own chain reaction of further problems.

You can see why, of the main pillars founding the new health system, knowledge has to be the fundamental one. For Robert Kowalski to cure his circulatory problem after orthodox medicine had failed, he had to know something about his condition. Other actions that are showing themselves to be important are reverting to Nature and to natural foods and products and concentrating on techniques that facilitate the elimination of the many toxins, dietary and environmental, with which our 20th-century bodies are becoming increasingly overloaded.

There is one other important factor in the new health equation – you. Your knowledge of yourself and how your body reacts, gained from observations over the years, is vital. One of the things we now recognize is that each person, each individual, is unique. What is medical sauce for the goose is not necessarily sauce for the gander. This is why some people seem to be able to get away with murder in their hectic, junk-food lifestyles, while others of us struggle just to stay on top.

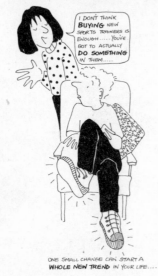

ONE SMALL CHANGE CAN START A **WHOLE NEW TREND** IN YOUR LIFE....

There is no justice when it comes to health, only trial, error, and finally, deserved better health. Through this process you can build up a knowledge of yourself which is second to none.

Remember, knowledge about health is not an exclusive club which can only be joined by the qualified. What are qualifications anyway, but crystallizations of knowledge acquired at a time which may well have become superseded by more recent findings?

We are in a period now when discoveries are being made at such a rate that they would defy any doctor busily occupied in treating the sick to keep up with them all.

In these circumstances, investigatory health writers and researchers such as myself can bridge the gap and provide an interim service manual such as this. We are fortunate in that our job has enabled us to travel the world and learn from some of the foremost thinkers of our time. The knowledge presented here is a distillation of their thoughts.

2

*

INTRODUCTION TO BODY-SYSTEMS MAINTENANCE

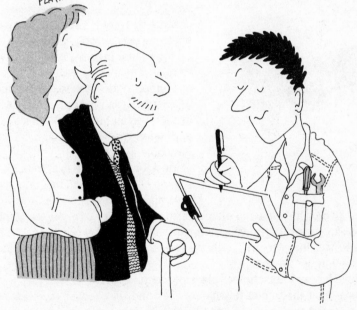

HE'D LIKE HIS **70-YEAR SERVICE** : OIL CHANGE, CHECK HIS WIRING, LUBRICATION OF ALL MOVING PARTS.... OH, AND HIS FUEL PUMP IS PLAYING UP A BIT.....

IN THIS CHAPTER

* Controlling the ageing process * Healthy systems maintenance * Picking up past threads * Stone-Age diet guidelines * Mal-health-practice checklist *v.* good-health-practice checklist * The Royal road to health

---

TURNING BACK THE CLOCK

Most of us are born healthy, with an innate sense of body balance and harmony. One only has to see the way a baby placed on the floor sits, back perfectly straight, to know that posture, a vital aspect of health, is inborn. One only has to watch the way a child leaps out of bed in the morning to know that energy, life energy, flows from a clear and seemingly endless fountain in youth.

Yet somehow that perfect posture deteriorates into slumping and stooping as we get older; like newly-planted trees we shoot up straight as saplings but afterwards become bent and gnarled in response to our environment. Limbs stiffen, and the wonderful springs of energy get

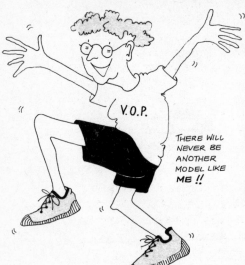

V.O.P.

THERE WILL NEVER BE ANOTHER MODEL LIKE ME !!

blocked. A feature of the old is their immobility, their stiffness, and the process by which it happens is called ageing.

Ageing is an important word when we think of health, because it describes a process we are going to try to reverse. If only we could stay on top of that process, keep the body flexible and moving and able to act as a good conductor to the sources of energy within it, we could maybe live forever. In fact some seers, yogis and wise men from the East, say we could.

Most of us would not want that, but we certainly would be content to live an active threescore and ten

years, free of the clogging effects of the passage of time on our joints, muscles, arteries, digestive systems and brains. And modern health science tells us that we can, if only we would do a bit of body maintenance on the way to old age.

Consider our cars, another piece of machinery we use. We recognize full well that they need regular services and oil changes to clean out accumulated sludge, otherwise they would soon seize up and the moving parts wouldn't move anymore. We also know that they need specialized fuel. Yet we happily go on expecting our bodies to run for life without any kind of overhaul, and on whatever fuel we fancy drinking and eating. We can get a new model car; we cannot get a new model body. And the spare parts business is pretty dicey.

Machines are made up of systems: the car and body are no exceptions. Each has a fuel system, a wiring system, a moving parts system and a lubrication system. Where the body differs is that it has a self-repair system which is little short of miraculous. But it is not infallible; repairs are done only when no other (or minimal) demands are being made on the body, such as during sleep. Which is why sound sleep is so important, but more of that later.

To return to the car and the body; in every system there is a weak point, an Achilles' heel, some part that needs special care. Every car buff, every car mechanic, will tell you that certain models of car are significant for their inherent faults, as well as for their good points. These are the points that need special care, special maintenance.

In bodies there are often inherited weaknesses, conditions that run in families. Sometimes they are more physical in their effects; sometimes they are more mental, more to do with temperament. This last factor introduces a dimension that doesn't exist in cars and other domestic machinery – call it the human factor. (Some car buffs would disagree with me, they think cars are temperamental too.)

What are we getting at? We are getting at the fact that the body can be likened to a car, a piece of machinery we use, and that we could well take a leaf out of our book of treating the car, and apply it to our bodies – regular servicing, careful monitoring of fuel, keeping the moving parts lubricated, etc. But that is not all: there are subtle differences between the car and the body and these we must take into account.

1. The body has to last us for life.
2. The body, if given half a chance, is self-repairing, even of serious conditions – provided it has the necessary spare parts to effect the repair. We must provide these in the fuel (food, water, etc.) we put into the system and the maintenance (therapy, lifestyle, etc.) we select.
3. Because you cannot take the body apart and peer into it as you can a car, you need to be aware of its main systems and, more importantly, of its symptoms. A stitch in time saves nine.

Systems and *symptoms*: here lies the double-sided key to understanding your body. The other part of the equation, call it the lock into which the key fits, is the *maintenance manual*. So there it is: systems, symptoms, maintenance manual – what could be simpler?

Remember, you already have a very big ace up your sleeve in the body itself: it knows how to repair every one of its systems; you need only provide it with a nudge in the right direction – plus the appropriate set of circumstances, or environment, in which to effect the repair. And that – the *right environment or conditions* – is the fourth and final factor of successful maintenance.

This fourth factor can be explained by referring once more to car maintenance. If you want to repair your car, you don't hang out of the

9

window while you are driving along the motorway and attempt to jiggle under the bonnet, should your arms be long enough. You have to take it to a repair shop where it remains until the repair is effected – you know that to your cost.

So it is with the body, or should be. The body favours resting repairs, not running repairs. But the fact is, what we've been doing to our bodies in the latter part of the 20th century is no body's business. We have been getting away with murder – think about that – we **are** murdering ourselves. And as we can see from the statistics quoted in Chapter 1 (about the number of people who are getting cancer and heart disease) we are starting to serve the sentence. It is not only our medical system that is failing us but our 20th-century lives. Our modern lifestyles and our habits have eroded the body's fabulous reserves of life, and now we are really in danger.

How has this happened? Car mechanics will tell you that, in order to put something right, you have to know what has gone wrong. We tend to think of our society as the golden age of scientific mastery, but what it really is turning into is gilded age of scientific misery. We have made ourselves sick by our modern lifestyles.

LEARNING FROM THE PAST

In the olden days, when most people worked outside in the fields, everybody got plenty of exercise, bending, stooping, pushing, pulling and walking miles to and from work because there was little or no transport. They also ate food grown naturally in the fields – no frozen food, no fast food, no packaged or tinned food, no need to buy a copy of *E for Additives* to see what had been added in the way of chemicals. What they ate may have been limited, but it was natural. At night, when they slept – and there was no city noise, electric light or television to keep them awake way past their natural bedtime – they slept, usually the sleep of the dead because they were so dog-tired from all that physical exercise. No sleeping pills.

Even the ale they drank was brewed naturally, and still contained much of the goodness of the grain. If they consumed pleasure foods such as ice-cream (and only on high days and holidays could they afford to go through the lengthy freezing process involved), it certainly was not made of pig fat or dried blood as most of it is today. Nor was white sugar added to it. Chocolate was virtually unheard of.

Yes, it was a hard life, but whoever said that a soft life was healthy? Yes, many people died of infections and confinements and dreadful accidents before their time, but they did live closer to nature and closer to each other, too. Today, we have a different set of diseases and conditions caused by a deficiency of Nature, and natural things, in our lives. We also have a deficiency of mutual support from each other.

Of course, everyone knows we cannot turn back the clock – and if we could we would lose much that we have gained from technology. But we can revert to some of the ways that, in retrospect, have been shown to be much healthier for us than before, with a few updatings.

In this way we can learn from the past. Keep in mind that the body has been around for half a million years more than modern convenience foods have – and these, incidentally, have thrown the human body the biggest curved ball of its historical evolvement. The digestive processes that were developed through the Stone Age simply have not caught up with modern food options: they are still happier with the fruit, nuts, berries, grain and occasionally fish and meat (when they could be caught) that were available to eat then, most of which was eaten raw. This is why a return to that kind of diet always improves vitality.

So is that what we are advocating – a return to munching apples in the Garden of Eden? Not at all; if we did that we would feel unspeakably cramped and uncomfortable – a bit like trying to live in an old movie. No; we must not go round in circles, we must ascend in a spiral, taking the best of the past with us, and sifting and discarding what it is of the present that is making us ill.

And we have to clean up our environment too. Gaia, as some people like to call the Earth, needs to be returned to health if she is to support us in our endeavours instead of making our task more difficult through pollution, etc. She is the bottom line of our environment, and just as health must become the responsibility of the individual in our new age scheme of things, so must looking after Gaia.

Returning once more to the art of car maintenance in order to follow its guidelines for body maintenance, we must now take a leaf out of the garage mechanic's book and formulate a good-practice checklist for the body, which we must quickly substitute for the malpractice checklist we have all inadvertently been following. Cast your pencil over the following, and see how many of the items apply to you.

11

MALPRACTICE CHECKLIST

1. Poor diet: food chosen for convenience or comfort rather than for health.
2. Drinking the wrong things, including tap water (especially when it is drunk iced with meals, which slows down the digestive process, which functions best at blood temperature).
3. Inadequate rest.
4. Inadequate exercise.
5. Disturbed breathing rhythm (sighing, shallow breathing, sharp intakes of breath) or breathing impure air.
6. Feelings of hopeless/helplessness; life lacks meaning.
7. Not enough balance between work and play.
8. Unsatisfactory relationships/absence of appreciation.
9. Increasing inability to handle stress.

Of those nine points, the last four of which are really lifestyle problems and therefore more difficult to resolve, do you know that it may be necessary to change only **one** to bring about an amazing transformation in vitality levels? This in turn will have a positive effect on any lifestyle problems you may have, because they will seem easier to tackle.

Sounds like a pipe-dream? Not so many years ago, if somebody had suggested that we could send a document down a telephone line, people would have laughed. Now we take facsimile (fax) for granted. Not so very long ago people were dying in droves from a variety of infections. Now we have antibiotics, and although they are a two-edged sword not to be abused, they have dramatically reduced deaths from infections.

Not so very long ago, doctors did not study nutrition at all in medical school; now that its extreme importance to health is recognized, it is being incorporated and will benefit future generations enormously. Meanwhile, since the whole point of this book is that we can't wait, here is a good-practice checklist.

GOOD-PRACTICE CHECKLIST

1. Fresh food diet: living food makes living bodies livelier.
2. Drinking pure liquids not full of poisoning additives.
3. Better sleep and rest, through learning simple techniques.
4. Quick, easy and non-boring exercise tips.
5. Diaphragm breathing techniques to clean out gassy poisons, and other clean out techniques for the fuel and energy systems.
(Remember, ageing is synonymous with clogging and stagnation.)
6, 7, 8 and 9. Tender loving care – A vital ingredient that the body simply cannot live without. (Car buffs would assure me that their cars need it too.)

From the good-practice checklist we can now derive the formula for health, and here it is. Let your **symptoms** guide you to locate your body **systems** that need overhaul; find the place in your **mainten-ance manual** and proceed with the repair, preferably in the right **environmental conditions**. This could also be expressed as: 1. Symptoms → 2. Systems → 3. Maintenance manual → 4. Repair and prevention procedures → 5. Health!

Note that inherent in the maintenance and repair procedures described in this book are prevention procedures – you don't clear your car of rust without applying rust inhibitors to stop it from happening again.

If you follow these procedures well you can keep your body healthy until you are ready to die. Indeed, future generations may even be able to do as yogis suggest, and choose the day!

3

❋

YOUR SYMPTOMS: GUIDE TO THE SYSTEMS

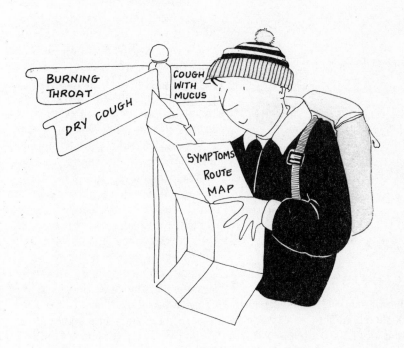

IN THIS CHAPTER

❋ Symptoms – signposts to discovery ❋ Systems – signposts to health ❋ Why illness is of value ❋ The subtle spectrum of health ❋ Diseases of our time ❋ Waking (and wising) up

Before you start turning to the chapters on the systems of the body, pause a moment. You may think you know which chapters are relevant to you, and you probably do, but put your body to the acid test by doing a symptoms checklist as described in this chapter first.

One of the keys to understanding all your body systems and how well they are working in connection with your lifestyle is to be found in noting your symptoms. Symptoms, however minor, are vital signposts to health.

It is important to start recording symptoms that happened in childhood, even babyhood. Remembering your early symptoms and keeping a careful record of those of your family is one of the most valuable health exercises you can undertake.

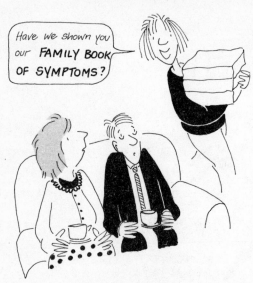

Orthodox medicine has not entirely realized the tremendous importance of symptoms – something that homoeopathic medicine has always understood. Homoeopathy is based on recording every single flicker of a symptom, and its remedies are fine-tuned by considering all of them in relation to each other.

Do not just note your symptoms: note how, when and under what circumstances they manifest themselves. However slight, however small, however seemingly unconnected, these little coincidences are the red flags that your system puts out to signify what is going wrong.

Until you get to the bottom of those, you may not entirely know which of the nine body systems described will be of special importance to you – apart, that is, from the sections on diet (see Chapter 4), the absorption and elimination of food and drink (see Chapters 4 and 10) and nutrition (Chapter 4). These factors are so fundamental to health and so often taken for granted as to be of importance to everyone. Diet – which does not mean eating less food – is the linchpin of health. This we now know.

Here are some spare lines and suggested headings under which you can jot down the key words of your symptoms. Or make your own headings. While you are doing this, make symptom sheets for the rest of the family to keep in the book. You may even wish to extend this to a big family tree of symptoms.

Don't omit symptoms that are to do with mood, vitality and so on, because you will discover that they may relate to under- or over-activity in some organs of your body, and they are often directly connected to lifestyle problems.

Use pencil! You may come back later to find your symptoms have disappeared – or changed direction!

Don't be ashamed of recording your symptoms, even the embarrassing ones like wind or bad breath or an itchy bottom! If you're frightened someone might pick up this book and know you all too well, give each family member a code name or number.

SYMPTOM CATEGORIZER

Family member:

Symptom:

Description:

Frequency/incidence:

History (when it started):

Family history (of similar symptoms):

Triggers (to your system):

Special comments:

PINNING DOWN YOUR SYMPTOMS

Did you have trouble describing your symptoms in a few key words? If you did, that's good: if you didn't, now is the time to think more deeply about them. Stomach aches, for example, take many forms: they can be localized and stabbing, turbulent and cramp-like, or gnawing, like excessive hunger-pangs. Coughs can be dry and rasping, moist and rattling, continuous or sporadic, prompted by cold or by wind or by a certain stress. The permutations are certainly vast, but not endless.

It may be worth while getting a separate piece of paper and writing down a fuller description of your symptoms, after your first attempt, but for the time being, for those urgent souls who want to press on, here is an interesting thought.

Although annoying in themselves, your symptoms exist not to annoy you but to attract your attention.

Symptoms are the symbols of our illness or complaint, whether they are mental, physical or a combination of the two. They are as graphic as a painting or a picture, they are a language that never lies.

Most people's symptoms are a mixture of the physical and the mental. For example, when you get a pain in your back (physical), you may feel tired and tearful, or tired and testy (mental, emotional). When you get indigestion (physical) you may feel uptight (mental, emotional) or fed up (think about that!). When you get PMT, you may feel bloated and suicidal or you may feel hyperactive and murderous. (There are actually four different categories of PMT, all with special recourses; see Chapter 9.)

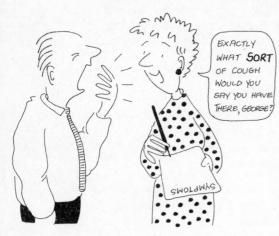

Which comes first: the chicken of the physical symptom or the egg of the emotional symptom? That's an important thing to record, but both types of symptom will be important in helping you and your new-age doctor gauge what is wrong with you and what remedy, or course of treatment, to suggest.

So many people suppress their mental and emotional symptoms because they feel guilty about them or because they think they are a sign of weakness. So you don't tell: you bottle them all up and, of course, they get worse! (Symptoms, like mothers-in-law, have a habit of upping the ante on you when you don't acknowledge them).

SIGNPOSTING FROM YOUR SYMPTOMS

Once you have located the source of most of your symptoms, you will find that the chapter headings and short introductory lists will help to guide you towards the sections that you want to read. Having done that, of course, you will want to start thinking about the measures you will take – diet, remedies, therapies and so on. There is a short appendix of useful addresses at the back of the book, including nutritional suppliers and helpful organizations, to guide your initial enquiries.

Nine body systems have been described here (it is amazing how much disagreement there is among experts as to how many systems the body actually has!) but the last, the secret, or energy system, is the most exciting. Obscured and unrecognized for many years, it is now attracting the most attention and research. So you may like to read about it for interest's sake, because it looks like becoming as important as the digestive system, perhaps more, since the energy system secretly controls all other systems.

As far as the remainder of the systems are concerned, if you are in any doubt which is relevant to you, ask a member of your family what they think you should read – 'Do I have PMT badly enough to affect family relationships?' 'Do I need to read the sections on stress in the nervous system chapter, even though I think I've got it under control?'

One other point I should mention is that this book is not a substitute for diagnosis by your doctor. There is no formula for diagnosing illnesses here – how could there be? There is merely information – knowledge – about new avenues of thought in health: new ways of approaching matters to do with your body, your health, your life.

Before moving on, here are a few more thought-provoking modern ideas for you to toss around in your mind:

● Illness is a symptom! Doubledutch? Not really. Illness is the ultimate symptom, and as such illness, any illness has a meaning.
● Illness is a sign that something is wrong with your life, and the nature of the illness will tell you what.

Let's look at a few popular sayings that may provide clues to the origins of an illness – that is, when, back in the dim and distant past, it may have started: 'She gets on my nerves . . . that woman is a pain in the neck . . . when I think of my driving test I get sick to the stomach . . . I can't shoulder that burden any longer . . . he's a thorn in my flesh . . . she gets under my skin . . . I feel as if I'm carrying the world on my back . . . that *galls* me . . . I can't get a grip on it . . . I could tear my hair out . . . you're a pain in the arse!'

Doctors 'in the know' have discovered that every organ in the body corresponds to an emotion as well as to a physical function.

HOW YOUR MIND GETS INTO YOUR BODY

Let's take an example of this link between mind and body. Most people recognize, at least subconsciously, the connection between the body's pump, the heart, and love. These are once again expressed in our language by such sayings as 'my heart bleeds for you . . . eat your heart out, Valentine . . . have a heart (when you want someone to show you feeling) . . . it's a real heartache' and so on. People who have had heart surgery say that they often cry like babies afterwards, their feelings well up as never before.

It appears that we often get the symptom in the organ that corresponds to the emotion that we find hardest to express. It's as if the organ is shouting at us: ignore part of my function and I'll show you – I'll give you gyp!

This is not to suggest, of course, that people who have heart trouble are hard-hearted (an interesting description!). They may care a great deal, but they may find it hard to relate to or express the more tender side of their feelings. Or they may feel, even if it's not really so, thwarted or frustrated or let down in love. Isn't it interesting that men, who find it more difficult to show their feelings, are more prone to heart troubles than women, who traditionally **do** show their feelings?

The lungs are to do with taking up, breathing and embracing life, getting in touch with what life is all about (the breath of life), of being prepared to live life for all it's worth. When this drive is thwarted, sadness is often the result, revealed in distortions of breathing, such as sighing a lot, of taking in air sharply as do people when they've been crying. Sometimes, people with lung complaints try to work and reason all their problems out in their heads, or talk about them constantly, thus suppressing other ways of dealing with them.

The liver, the body's main chemical or metabolic plant, is to do with assimilating life and making something of it. If life heaps insults and disappointments on a person to the point where they feel they cannot take another setback or another disappointment, so that their will becomes paralysed, a liver condition may develop. It is well known that those who contract hepatitis experience great depression before the onset of the disease.

In the same vein, another manifestation of paralysed will can occur with arthritis. Arthritics have been described as people who have a lot of 'shoulds' and 'oughts' in their nature: they somehow have allowed life to 'cramp' their style.

Stomach complaints may be a sign of not being able to 'stomach' one's circumstances: the word 'dyspeptic', which has come to mean 'irritable', describes it perfectly. Only one step on from there, of course, is irritable bowel syndrome, which now afflicts something like 11 per cent of our population.

Skin complaints, if one considers the role of the skin as a barrier, suggest that the inner person is somehow being 'rubbed up the wrong way' by the environment.

Fascinating, isn't it, that who and what we are is not only expressed by what we do, or by our personalities, but by our complaints and illnesses too? The illness (or symptom) is substituting for the missing ingredient in life.

What should be emphasized is that there should be no suggestion of criticism of oneself or of others in displaying any symptom or contracting any illness. People are often unaware of the combined effects that diet, childhood, opportunity and circumstance have had on their lives; only by the manifestation of a symptom or, finally, the illness is the awareness brought into conscious focus, when it can be recognized and dealt with. Illness itself is the symptom.

Here is another thought-provoking 'discovery'. **Illness is a spectrum;** at one end of it is health, at the other, death.

How many people have visited their doctor with symptoms, to be told 'there's nothing organic' or 'there's nothing really wrong. Come back later'? And later, when you do go back, maybe even years later, there **is** often something wrong. You have progressed further along the spectrum away from wellness towards illness. Preventive medicine plans to tackle your problem when, like a leak in a hosepipe, it is only a small one. The above situation, no doubt familiar to many, is yet another reason for paying early attention to your symptoms and for seeking to alleviate them. When more serious symptoms show your doctor that your illness has progressed to a disease, it may be too late.

DISEASES OF OUR TIME

It is interesting to note that some diseases seem to be characteristic of the age in which we live; this is because the structure of society at any time is reflected in the illnesses of those who live in that society. When you think about it, we live in a society where the hard-headed mental qualities of thinking, learning, rationalism and realism, have dominated the softer hearted, more flexible qualities of feeling and intuition. Is it any wonder that one of our greatest killers is arterial disease or hardened arteries, affecting especially the head (strokes) and heart (heart attacks)? Yet another killer is cancer, whereby the suppression of chances to be creative and caring has led the body to create its own negative growth structure in their place. In the old days people used to bake cakes, make tools and equipment as well as mend and maintain things, but now those simple acts of creativity have been taken over by technology. Of course, this is just one aspect of a very complex set of causes and events: environmental and lifestyle factors have also contributed to weakening the body's defence systems against disease. For example, it has been estimated that the average person these days now ingests each year 1g (0.03oz) of lead and 4.5kg (10lb) of food additives, and has 4.5l (1 gallon) of pesticides sprayed on the fruit and vegetables they eat. Add to that our *sedentary* lifestyles (think about that word, linked by root to the noun sediment: it is the key to what is happening to the body) and you will begin to have some idea of just how much harder we have to work to be healthy. We can't just let it happen: we have to make it happen.

WAKING UP

Awareness is the first part of knowing. I hope that what follows will encourage you to perceive how easy it is to help your health. The body is truly miraculous: if given half the chance, it is self-repairing, even of serious conditions, as long as it has the necessary spare parts to effect the repair. We must provide these in the fuel (food, water, etc.) we put into the system and the maintenance (therapy, lifestyle, exercise, etc.) we select.

So, record your symptoms, even if they are things such as boredom, inertia, hopelessness or fatigue. If you have created them, you can create something more positive in their place.

One final note: when you are reading about the systems, you will find therapies are suggested from time to time that may be helpful to their function. However, actual recommendations are only rarely given: this is because the search for the right therapist should be as individual as the need that has created it. In the final analysis, it is the therapist who matters, not the therapy.

Most reliable therapists – not all – are members of groups or associations that set professional standards for their practitioners in order to protect the interests of patients. Looking at the small ads in a reliable health magazine or in the yellow pages under the name of the therapy is a good starting point, as is writing to the magazine, with a stamped, self-addressed return envelope, for advice.

4

*

THE ALL-IMPORTANT DIGESTIVE AND EVACUATION SYSTEM

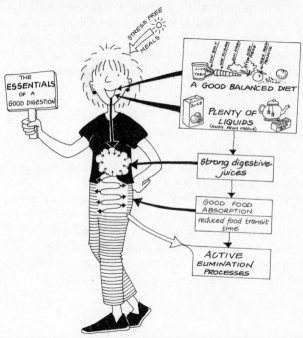

IN THIS CHAPTER

✻ System workings ✻ Conquering candida ✻ Understanding indigestion ✻ Luscious raw-food benefits ✻ Basic protein needs ✻ 12 tips for healthier digestion ✻ Choosing fast foods ✻ Slimming that works ✻ Energetic food combining ✻ Cooking the healthy way ✻ Why we need vitamins and amazing aminos ✻ Getting nutritional advice ✻ 10 golden rules of elimination ✻ Conquering constipation

You are what you eat . . . or are you? It's a well-known maxim but, like most maxims, it is only true under certain circumstances. Actually, you are what you can **absorb** of what you eat. However, the underlying meaning is true, because every cell in the body is constructed from the raw materials that we consume in the way of food and drink. Because of this, the system that digests this fuel and converts it, either into energy for life or into body structures, has a major bearing on health. Thus it is the single most important system, and the major linchpin of health.

Before reading on, conduct a little experiment on yourself. List, in the space provided below, the different foods you have eaten during the past week. Then list the different liquids you have drunk. Don't forget to include medications and medicines. List everything you have put into your mouth, even things you haven't swallowed, such as chewing gum. Later, when you know more about your choices, you will be able to analyse whether your intake is sound or not from information gleaned in this chapter and in Chapters 11 and 12, where we look at how what you eat affects the working of your immune system and your energy production system.

YOUR DIGESTIVE SYSTEM: HOW IT WORKS

A charming Irishman once sold me (on April Fool's Day) a complete set of *Encyclopaedia Britannica*. I have thanked heaven for it on many occasions. Looking it up – as I did – to discover more about the digestive system, I discovered these words: 'The digestive tract begins at the lips and ends at the anus.' Short and clear, but how many people pay attention to it? Most think the digestive tract ends at the stomach, the rest being just for getting rid of debris. In fact, matter is absorbed all the way down the intestines, and the fact that some medications are given rectally proves that even in the rectum, the last bit of the intestine before the anus, matter can be absorbed.

Keeping the system clear and able to utilize fully its fuel is of vast importance – just as important as it is to keep the fuel and oil lines of your car unclogged. And while it is readily accepted that cars run on only the purest fuel and need regular oil changes to keep their systems clear, few people recognize the importance of similar needs for the body. Yet there are some wonderful ways of cleansing the digestive system, which will be discussed later.

THE DIGESTIVE PROCESS

Over the lips, over the gums . . . look out stomach, here it comes! And so it does: swallowed food plummets straight into the stomach, dropping at the incredible speed of 7.6m (25ft) a second! Once there the process of digestion gets going in earnest, as food is mixed with powerful gastric juices by the strongly muscular churning action of the stomach.

However, the initial process of digestion really begins in the mouth, where, by the action of chewing, food combines with saliva, which contains complex enzymes that start the digestive processes. Chewing food thoroughly is important in order to mix in these enzymes, so chew, chew, chew, chew, chew, chew and chew: food should be nearly liquid by the time it reaches the stomach.

Stomach acid, the next digestive aid, is infinitely more powerful than saliva. One of its main constituents is hydrochloric acid, and it is extremely strong, as anyone who has ever vomited will know! Having strong stomach acid is vital for digestion. However after the age of 40, the stomach's ability to produce hydrochloric acid diminishes significantly, and by middle age it has been reduced by about 50 per cent, which explains why the cast-iron digestions of the young are so different from the more delicate digestions of the older generation. This has to be taken into account in the diet.

Fortunately, there are ways to supplement this shortfall, since there are natural means by which the stomach may be encouraged to produce more acid, such as by eating very finely chopped, raw mild onion – considered indigestible by many, in fact, given time, it has exactly the reverse effect!

Depending on the mixture of food, the stomach will usually empty its contents in two to five hours, by which time food has become a semi-fluid mass called chyme. This passes through the pylorus sphincter (or valve) into the duodenum to begin its journey through the intestines, which incredibly, are nearly 8m (over 25ft) long (that's longer than most people's gardens).

The internal surface area of the intestines that is available for absorption is estimated by some experts (such as those of *Encyclopaedia Britannica*) to be an incredible 4,500 square metres (or if you prefer to be astounded in yards, 5,400 square yards)! Others are more conservative (it is amazing how much disagreement there is on the body) and suggest the absorbing area is about the size of a tennis court (260 sq m/310 sq yd). In any case, this should cope with most square meals! Hair-like protuberances, called villi, on the surface of the intestines help to achieve this amazing surface area. A cross-section of them would look like a section through a deep-pile carpet.

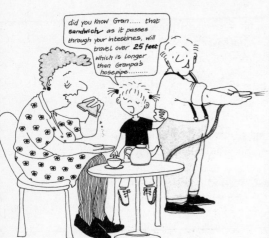

DUODENUM

The duodenum, or first part of the intestine, is extremely important. Most people have heard of it, because it is frequently a place where people get ulcers. Although it is less than 30cm (1ft) of the entire intestinal length, it contains the electrical 'pacemaker' that regulates the speed at which food moves through the small intestine; it is also the area that receives further digestive juices from the liver and from the pancreas. Many dozens of catalysts such as enzymes are employed by the body to digest the food we eat, some of which are contained in bile from the liver, and others from pancreatic juices.

THE LIVER: GIVER OF LIFE

Everything we digest goes through the liver. This magnificent organ, one of the body's largest and weighing 1.5–2kg (3–4lb), is a veritable chemical factory, with literally hundreds of vital duties. It processes all fat, manufacturing bile to aid its digestion, which is stored in the gall bladder for ready use when high-fat meals are consumed (as they all-too-frequently are in Western diets).

The liver also filters and cleans the blood of waste matter, poisons such as alcohol and nicotine, drugs, industrial chemicals, additives and so on. It changes sugar into insoluble glycogen so that it can be stored out of the bloodstream where it would otherwise do harm, and changes it back again when fuel is needed. It breaks down the nitrogen in food to urea so that the kidneys can process it (this is an example of organs working together, which is why their functions can never be separated, one from the other, as orthodox medicine has tried to do). As if this were not enough, it also balances the sex hormones and regulates blood clotting. Thank heavens it can regenerate itself given rest and moderate eating habits. It is the only organ that can.

THE PANCREAS AND INSULIN

The pancreas is another vital organ of which people will have heard, since it secretes insulin, without which sugar diabetes occurs. Diabetes is a classic example of just how serious it can be if just one of the vital digestive substances is not being produced in the body. However the pancreas produces far more than insulin, which is part of its **endocrine** function (see Chapter 9). It also has an **exocrine** function, secreting many digestive enzymes directly into the intestines, without which the best diet in the world would simply not be assimilated.

The next part of the intestine (from the duodenum) is called the jejunum, where fats are absorbed, and some people have this part shortened surgically when they absorb too many fats. (The things we have done to us!) After that, food passes into the ileum and then the colon, the latter being another familiar term. Actually the colon is better known as the large intestine because of its larger diameter, and it is there that the liquid 'food' becomes more solid, due to the reabsorption of water, in preparation for faeces to be formed and passed out through the anus. The colon can be a frequent source of health problems, because food often lies about stagnating in it for far too long (see below).

OUR PRECIOUS INTESTINAL FLORA

It is in the colon that the final absorption of minerals and the disintegration of food residue occurs, and this is done with the help of intestinal parasites, generally known as flora, which consist of bacteria, yeasts and fungi. The colon has been called our 'earth', and just as the earth of the garden needs worms and parasites to help it break down the minerals and make them accessible to growing plants, so we need parasites to help us with digestion. Most people find it amazing to learn that they have more than 1.5kg (2–3lb) of these parasites active in their intestines at any given time.

These flora must be kept in balance with each other, and everyone knows what happens when antibiotics are taken and the helpful bacterial parasites get killed along with the harmful bacterial infection we are fighting. The result is gas, discomfort, indigestion, constipation or diarrhoea, thorough misery and what doctors often call an irritable bowel. Which is why fresh, **live** yoghurt (not flavoured or sweetened) should be taken with antibiotics to replace the good parasites that have been lost. Better still, take acidophilus powder, since acidophilus is one of the strains of beneficial flora present in the gut that is depleted by antibiotics. Both 'live' yoghurt and acidophilus powder are available from health food stores. Look for powder that contains bifidus as well and has to be refrigerated, as the rest of the products on the market are of lesser strength. (Perfectionists take each strain separately and alternately on an annual basis: one month acidophilus, one month bifidus, one month bulgaricus, then rest for 6 – 9 months, unless antibiotics are taken in that period.)

Another well-known saying about the colon has not such a pleasant ring. It is that 'death begins in the colon'. Never forget this. By the time food reaches the colon or large intestine, it has already been in the gut for 8–10 hours, and it is undergoing a process of putrefaction and decay similar to that which occurs in a compost heap (although not as healthy). Since the food is likely to remain in the colon for another 24 hours at least, it is not surprising that it often smells so rotten – frequently it **is** rotten! The intestinal bacteria have incompletely broken down what is left of the food into 'manure'. This may be very good for gardens, but it is not so good for intestines, especially as many of us have unhealthy, leaky intestinal linings, which allow the compost/manure to leak into the bloodstream where it is recognized as poison. This our immune system, kidneys and liver have to detoxify, thus augmenting their load. No wonder overworked livers are a common feature of our times, and the underlying cause of many chronic conditions such as candidasis.

CANDIDA OVERGROWTH: A 20th CENTURY DISEASE

It is unhealthy intestinal flora overgrowth which renders the gut leaky. The name candida (thrush) has become **the** 20th-century complaint. Most ME sufferers have it, and most cancer sufferers have it, but many so-called healthy people have it as well without realizing, although an itchy bottom or frequently occurring attacks of mouth or vaginal thrush are often signs. It can be the precursor of many more serious illnesses because it overworks the body's defence systems, leaving them weakened and unable to cope with their real work of defending the system from foreign invaders and from cancer.

Candida overmultiplies under certain circumstances – such as on a high-sugar or junk-food diet or during a course of antibiotics (the contraceptive pill is also a factor) – and then it can change from the relatively harmless yeast form to a much more invasive fungal form, during which roots develop that actually penetrate the colon walls. It then dumps its toxins and waste products from its own digestive processes into our bloodstream, as well as allowing putrefactive matter from our own digestive processes through the breached colon walls – not a pretty picture.

It is easy to see how a continuous process like this can begin to undermine health. Unfortunately, we need some candida in our colons to help break down certain digestive wastes, so we cannot take a remedy which eliminates it entirely. But keeping it under control is vital. Remember that candida (commonly called thrush) is a form of yeast, and anyone who has ever seen yeast cause bread to rise in a matter of an hour knows how quickly it can multiply. Yeast loves sugar, and so anyone with thrush problems should eliminate sugar and all yeast-based and fermented products, including bread, alcohol, vinegar and marmite, from their diet for a time and eat plenty of roughage and vegetables. 'Fungal' foods such as mushrooms and mouldy cheese should also be omitted. There are many good books on candida and thrush available, and anyone who thinks they have a problem should scan the shelves of their specialist/health bookshop.

THE ALL-IMPORTANT TRANSIT-TIME OF FOOD IN THE INTESTINES

One solution to the above putrefactive dilemma is to try to cut down the transit time that food spends in the intestine so that there is less time for it to go rotten, which is why an all-vegetarian diet is so much healthier for us, because vegetables are far more quickly digested and expelled. It is meat/animal protein which largely causes the putrefaction in the colon. Dogs, which are almost exclusively meat-eaters, provide a classic example of just what kind of putrefaction meat-eating promotes!

Gut transit-time is only 36 hours for vegetarians compared with 72 hours for meat-eaters. It is terribly important for meat-eaters to eat plenty of fresh vegetables and fruit, because they contain bulk in the form of fibre and hence hurry things along. Wheat bran does the same thing but not as healthily, since it leaches out valuable minerals the body needs in the process. Contrary to popular belief, wheat bran is not particularly good for you. Other brans – such as rice bran and oat bran or psyllium husks – are better, and better still is the fibre found naturally in vegetables and salads.

THE FINAL STAGE OF EVACUATION

Finally, what is left of the food gets passed into the rectum and out. The more liquid we drink the softer, and easier, this process becomes. A liquid diet of alcohol does not help in this respect, unfortunately, because alcohol dries out the system (the raging hangover thirst bears witness to this), so it is other forms of liquid that we must look to for assistance.

The important thing to realize is that the colon must be kept as healthy and sweet as possible. It has to last us for a lifetime of digestion, and as dried-out, undigested food accumulates over the years, it frequently develops tarry deposits, which cling to the walls and slow down the peristalsis, the muscular movements that push food through the digestive tract. No wonder our colons get sluggish and baggy as we get older, and eventually the colon cells themselves become unhealthy and begin to die. Death, our death, really does begin in the colon, and we must do our best to delay this process, otherwise we will get less and less benefit but more and more toxins from the food we eat. The later section on elimination includes some suggestions and treatments for restoring the colon to its original healthy state. Recalling the earlier maxim we can now add: *we are what we eat and what we can absorb*. The colon is the vital second part of this equation.

THE ESSENTIALS OF GOOD DIGESTION

1. A good diet, consisting of plenty of fresh food and roughage.
2. Strong digestive juices, which themselves depend on good nutrition (see later).
3. Good absorption of food, which depends on having healthy linings to the intestinal walls and on all the right enzymes working together.
4. An active elimination process (for reasons mentioned above).

If the system breaks down anywhere, digestion is incomplete. And it is a vicious circle, because if digestion is incomplete, the raw materials the body needs, such as enzymes for digestion, simply cannot be manufactured. Without them, the digestion weakens further, and so on, down the slippery slope to ill health.

STRESS AND INDIGESTION: COMMON CURSES OF OUR AGE

There is one other powerful factor that adversely affects the digestive processes, and that is stress. The digestive juices are secreted – or in reverse dried up – by a part of the nervous system that is not under our conscious control.

Anyone who has ever salivated at the sight or smell of a delicious meal will know that this is a process which is quite involuntary. It is called the 'Pavlov's dog syndrome'. Unfortunately, the reverse effect – the digestive juices drying up – is also quite involuntary. If anything upsets us at mealtimes the digestive juices shut down, and the food remains in the stomach undigested for hours, or until the stress passes. This is why it is unwise to eat when stressed or upset, as indigestion will occur.

DO YOU REALLY NEED THAT INDIGESTION TABLET?

People tend to take antacid tablets for indigestion. Except for those few people who do produce too much stomach acid (most of us don't produce enough), this can be the worst possible measure. It is always important to establish the cause of indigestion, especially as producing too much acid can be the forerunner to an ulcer.

In most cases, indigestion is made worse by taking antacids, because acids are needed to digest the food in the first place. A far better recourse, having established that the cause of indigestion is not over-production of acid, is to take digestive enzymes in capsule form when you know you are going to tax your digestion with a heavy meal – especially if over forty! Remember this maxim: 40+ is digestive enzyme time. Three popular preparations are pineapple bromelain, papaya or betaine hydrochloride (especially for digesting protein). Some of these digestive aids are to be found naturally in fresh fruit, such as pineapple, papaya and apples – however stewing or cooking the fruit kills them, as they are living substances and are killed by heat.

The above is a preventive measure, but a quick cure for indigestion, once it has already set in, is to put four or five drops of peppermint essence (most good chemists stock it) into a small sherry glass of hot water and drink it down. (My aunt always used to take crème de menthe for this reason – or so she said.)

YOUR INDIGESTION GUIDE

For those who were fascinated by the link between emotions and their effects on the organs of the body as described in Chapter 3, here is a guide as to whether the origins of your indigestion are likely to be causing your gastric juices to shut down or to overproduce.

Fear, anger and frustration inhibit the flow of acid, but *chronic* anxiety increases it.

HOW RAW FOOD PROTECTS YOUR DIGESTION

The body does not like cooked food. In fact, it actually makes antibodies against it, in much the same way as it makes antibodies against cold and flu germs. The secret is to have a little fresh food before every cooked meal – a piece of carrot, a salad, some crudités. These raw foods persuade the body to relax its vigilance.

Knowing these things about the digestive process makes eating sensibly so much more logical. It is not just a fad, something cranky people do, but a genuinely wise move. This does not mean that all favourite foods have to be given up; simply that they should comprise *less* of the daily diet than before.

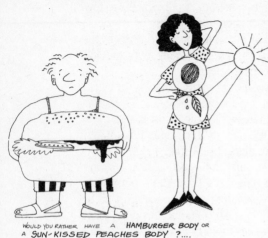

WOULD YOU RATHER HAVE A *HAMBURGER BODY* OR A *SUN-KISSED PEACHES BODY* ?....

HOW MUCH MEAT DO WE NEED?

Another way of tackling the problem of putrefaction, which can be so embarrassing and uncomfortable, since it produces smelly wind, is to eat less protein.

Apparently we need a lot less protein than was originally believed; in fact there is an equation which tells you exactly how much protein you need, either in the form of vegetable protein, such as beans and pulses, or of animal protein, such as meat, fish, eggs, cheese, in order to stay healthy. Here is that equation: 1 gram (0.03oz) of protein is required for every 1kg (2.2lb) of body weight. Growing children will require as much as four to five times this amount; vigorous exercisers will require at least half as much again.

For adults, this is a *ridiculously* small amount of protein: 100-150g (4 or 5oz) a day, much less than most people eat. Because meat is one of our most expensive food items and also one of our most polluted (animals consume fertilizers and are fed antibiotics and hormones), it can clearly be seen that a sensible diet is also likely to save money. The cost of good organic fresh vegetables and fruit will offset this only slightly.

But stop a minute. Answer this question: would you rather have a hamburger body or a sun-kissed peaches body?

It's a persuasive argument: if your diet consists of hamburgers and chips and fizzy drinks and coffee and sausages and fish fingers and pizzas and sandwiches and sweets and cans of instant soup and potato crisps and buns and pies, you are going to have a very different kind of body from a body constructed, say, of fresh fruit, salads, cereals, wholemeal bread, vegetables, lean meat and fish, and plenty of pure water. It is going to smell different, too. (An extreme example of this is perceived in the way an alcoholic smells when passed in the street – not all of it is grime!)

Now think of the smell of a fresh peach just picked off a tree . . . of strawberries, oranges, lemon zest . . . walk past a fruit and vegetable stall and smell the produce. Do you want a fresh peach body or a hamburger and chips body? It's never too late to change, because no cell in the body lives longer than seven years – all are reconstructed from the raw materials we eat.

There are additional reasons for favouring unprocessed (which means as fresh as possible) food. Food of this nature contains live information, because it is alive. So it adds life to your life, giving you a head start on those who eat only dead food. Horrible as it may seem, in the wild most things are eaten alive. And we come from the wild (stone age), which is why our digestive systems are still 'savage' in their construction. Ideally, 50-75 per cent of the food we eat should be raw.

HOMO NOT-SO-SAPIENS AND HIS MODERN NOT-SO-HEALTHY DIET

When you consider that our species *Homo sapiens* has been around for more than half a million years, it is not surprising that the last half century, a mere 50 years, has had little effect on the structure and functioning of our digestive systems. Archaeologists have discovered that during that time we ate mainly fruit, seeds and nuts and drank only pure water. Meat and fish were sparse adjuncts to the diet, grain was only added when we started to settle in one place, fewer than 10,000 years ago.

Our alimentary tracts have not changed since then, but our diets have, especially in the past two decades or so, when inventions such as freezers, microwaves and food irradiation have made it so easy for us to consume convenience food rather than prepare it in old-fashioned, time-consuming ways.

Fortunately, there is a swing back to food which is also fresh and pure – 'pure' meaning as unadulterated as possible – partly because it has now been shown beyond all doubt that nearly every ailment is considerably helped by a fresh food diet (see later).

So much for the digestive system – and 'much' is the operative word. The view presented here is very simplified, but it may help to reveal the magic which the body works and re-works every day as it digests our three meals for us and the literally thousands of complex chemical processes that are implemented – all of which are dependent on what we eat for their raw materials or spare parts. And the wondrous end-result? Energy for life. Your life and my life. Food is the fuel of life, and the better the digestion – that is, the better the furnace – the better the life. So to sum up, here are the:

TWELVE GOLDEN RULES OF HEALTHY DIGESTION

1. Avoid drinking tap water. Your area's water may be the exception to the more general rule that there are now too many chemicals and pollutants in tap water, but it is unlikely, so why take the risk? Drink 2 litres (at least 4 pints) of bottled, purified or distilled water a day, preferably apart from meals, otherwise digestive juices get diluted. Most chemists sell purified water in 5-litre (1 gallon) containers, which work out cheaper than buying bottles; or buy a *real* water purifier or distiller (see useful addresses), which works out cheaper still. Water-filtering jugs don't do the job well enough, although they do help, as long as you change the filter often enough – which you won't.

2. Limit the amount of fast foods that you eat. These foods contain far too much salt and fat, both of which are bad for you – very bad. If you must eat fast food at lunch time, leave the batter and the coatings or have vegetarian sandwiches, and steer clear of coloured and fizzy soft drinks even if they do not contain sugar. None of them is good for you – favour fruit juice or water. For between-meal treats have a piece of fruit or a fruity/cereal bar. Substitute carob for chocolate, or choose a chocolate that contains at least 60 per cent cocoa and little sugar.

3. Reduce your overall consumption of sugar and refined carbohydrates. This includes sweets, cakes, biscuits, crisps, jam, buns and white bread (up to 30 additives are present in the latter). If you have a sweet tooth and can't resist sweets or chocolates, always have them after a meal. Their bad effects are reduced at this time because the sugar they contain is not dumped directly into the bloodstream; and also there are more vitamins from your meal present in the body to help digest sugar's empty calories. Mums were right when they said no pudding until you've eaten your greens.

4. Reduce animal fat intake, especially of dairy produce – it encourages thick mucus which clogs the system. (Homo

not-so-sapiens is the only species that continues to drink milk after weaning, and it's not even our own milk we drink, but that of an animal three times our size, with a formula designed accordingly! No wonder dairy food makes us fat.) Avoid fried foods, and if you must eat dairy products, try to stick to skimmed milk and low-fat cheese. Use butter and margarine sparingly, but butter is better for you than margarine because it contains fewer additives and is far more natural. Cold-pressed olive oil is best for cooking and salads.

5. Eat lots of *fresh* vegetables, salads and fruit. Vegetables should be lightly cooked or eaten raw. Buy a seed-sprouter and sprinkle sprouted seeds on salads and sandwiches (they are cheap, tasty, full of enzymes and can be grown on any windowsill).

6. Eat plenty of fibre, but not wheat bran. As one well-known nutritionist says, 'that's for horses.' It really does block the absorption of valuable minerals, especially zinc, and thereby can contribute to PMT. Eat oat bran instead of wheat bran, because it really is good for the intestines and blood vessels, and also wholemeal bread, beans, including baked beans (the low-sugar variety), high-fibre vegetables, such as artichokes, asparagus, cabbage and leeks, natural cereals and brown (not white) rice.

7. Avoid additives, smoked and artificially coloured foods. Look at the labels of foods and choose those with the fewest additives. The body regards these substances as poisons, as it does alcohol, which should be limited to two drinks a day, preferably of beer or *good* wine (cheap wine contains a hair-raising number of chemicals).

8. Limit your intake of salt. The best way is not to add it during cooking or at table. Not only does excess salt lead to high blood pressure, but it also interferes with the uptake of other valuable minerals the body needs.

9. Eat a varied diet. Eating the same foods often causes allergies to develop, and this is especially true for children. Many people are allergic to wheat, and how often do we eat that? Variety **is** the spice of life, especially in diets, and eating different foods will also help ensure that you are more likely to get all the nutrients you need.

10. Try to sit down to eat and take it slowly. And don't eat late at night if you want to lose weight – you may be burning the midnight oil but you won't be burning off so many calories, since you'll be asleep soon after.

11. Eat small breakfasts – try fresh fruit, yoghurt, stone-ground oat or millet porridge, or muesli with a few added sesame, sunflower, pumpkin or flax seeds for super-plus nutrition plus a spoonful or two of granulated lecithin to help control cholesterol levels. The Continentals got this right, and the English and Americans got it wrong: eating cooked breakfasts to give you energy is a fallacy. Your

energy comes from the previous day's meals. A large breakfast actually diverts the body from its valuable job of eliminating toxins from the day before, which it will do until midday if you don't overload it with more heavy food.

12. Have a 'mad' day every week or so when you indulge yourself with your pet culinary vice – chocolates, a few drinks, cakes, a special meal. 'A too strict regime is a wearisome malady', says Doris Grant, author of *Food Combining For Health*.

COMPROMISE SUGGESTIONS

O.K., we live in the real world and we have to go to work every day – or we have to sit in certain cafés and restaurants with our not-so-health-conscious friends and we don't want to be on a food crusade all the time. Here's how to cope.

MAKING TAKE-AWAYS WORK FOR YOU

It is no good turning a blind eye to the fact that 25 per cent of all money spent on food outside the home goes on take-aways. It is convenient in this busy world to treat yourself to a take-away while watching television or a video. As with fast food lunches, these are often full of salt and fat (two wicked additions, both cheap, so they're used a lot).

However the 'Ordinary Persons' of this world (I call you the VOPs of the new health movement) can begin to put pressure on take-away companies (who are making a fortune in fast food) by demanding (and choosing) more wholesome take-aways – by asking for salad with your chicken, or by choosing Chinese food that doesn't contain mostly rice, batter or fried noodles but does contain quickly cooked vegetables. (Remember that chow mein is often a euphemism for leftovers.)

Here are some extra guidelines. Always start with a salad and end with a piece of fruit. They will fill you up. Shish kebab and salad is one of the best choices, as is a simply cooked jacket potato with salad. If you must have potato chips, try to find a place which cuts them thickly so that you get more potato and less rancid oil. With more elaborate take-aways look for less sauce, more substance.

Try not to drink tea, coffee, beer, cola or fizzy orange with your take-away but a nicely presented mineral water.

MAKING SLIMMING DIETS WORK FOR YOU

There is a book entitled *Dieting Makes You Fat*, and there's more than an element of truth in that title. Most of us who diet to lose weight soon become familiar with the ever-increasing difficulty of losing weight no matter how little we eat.

This is because the body uses its fats to store the toxins that build up over the years because of poor diet, faulty elimination, stress, fatigue and so on. Because fat in the body is extremely inert (as sufferers from cellulite know to their cost), it is a perfect storehouse for toxins, keeping them well out of the way of the bloodstream, where, if they were to circulate, they would make us feel very ill indeed. It is the toxins in the bloodstream that are responsible for most of our 'off' days – those days when we just don't feel well – and, of course, for the morning after the night before. Hence any worthwhile diet has got to be an elimination diet as well as a reduction diet, i.e. its ingredients have to be pure enough to enable the body to eliminate its toxins, and with them the fat it has been holding onto to protect you from the effects of the toxins!

Raw food is ideal for this purpose, expecially if it is organically grown, because its own tissues will contain infinitely fewer toxins from fertilizers and other chemicals than would be the case with commercially grown fruits and vegetables. Raw foods contain a lot of stored water in their tissues, which is very pure, and as such it makes a wonderful solvent for toxins, in much the same way that distilled water will absorb much more

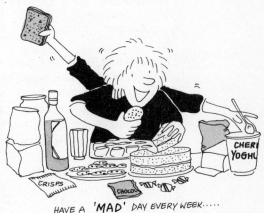

HAVE A 'MAD' DAY EVERY WEEK......

than tap water. The picture is more complex than that, but this is the general principle behind the modern reducing diet, which, surprisingly, does not so much count calories as count percentages of what you may eat – for example, 70 per cent of foods should be raw and high in water content and 30 per cent should be taken from such foods as whole grains, seeds, fish and game. Game is included because it is reared in the wild and not fed any of the polluting concoctions on which battery hens and commercially reared meat are raised. Lamb is also a good choice for this reason – its feed is natural grass.

This diet also depends on not eating anything but fresh fruit before midday, because the liver, the prime organ of detoxification, is most active between midnight and midday, and if anything but fruit is eaten during this period it diverts the liver once more to absorption, when elimination is what is wanted, especially your unwanted kilos of fat!

FOOD COMBINING: HOW TO HAVE YOUR CAKE, EAT IT AND STAY THIN!

Many people lose weight without dieting on this technique for eating. Nothing is banned in the way of food; how it is combined is the important factor.

The technique is based on the fact that proteins – meat, fish, cheese, eggs – are absorbed in a strongly acid medium, while carbohydrates are absorbed in a predominantly alkaline medium (the body produces digestive juices of both types). So, it is argued, if you mix the two types of food, they must both wait in the stomach and intestines until first one, then the other is digested. It is far better to eat one type of food at one meal, leave a gap of four hours, then eat the other at the next meal. Fortunately some foods are neutral and can be combined with either protein or carbohydrate. The diagram opposite shows what foods combine with what – yes, I'm afraid it does mean no hamburgers, no salmon bagels, no cheese with biscuits, no roast beef with Yorkshire pudding.

Because food is digested more easily in this way, people can lose weight without actually eating less. Furthermore, people who follow the principles of food combining say they have more energy, which also makes sense, because less energy is being diverted into digesting food. The title mentioned above by Doris Grant is an excellent book to buy for more detail and recipes, as are Harvey and Marilyn Diamond's books, such as *Fit for Life*.

COOKING FOOD THE ENERGETIC WAY

Now follows some advice on how to cook food to preserve its liveliness and freshness. This method was demonstrated by a clever scientist called Harry Oldfield, who has developed a photographic technique to enable us to see the energy field around food. (Every living thing has an energy field, which reflects the strength and nature of its energy – think of a magnet and the 'unseen' force around it and you will have an idea of what is meant).

The energy field around living objects is very beautiful – if you could see your own you would be transfixed by its swirling colours – and it is the appearance of this that tells us how healthy, how alive, we really are. (Read more about this in Chapter 12.) Food viewed in this way reveals its liveliness potential too. However, when such foods are cooked they lose much of their life-force and hence their goodness. Fortunately, some cooking techniques preserve it better than others. Here they are, in order of merit as they appear

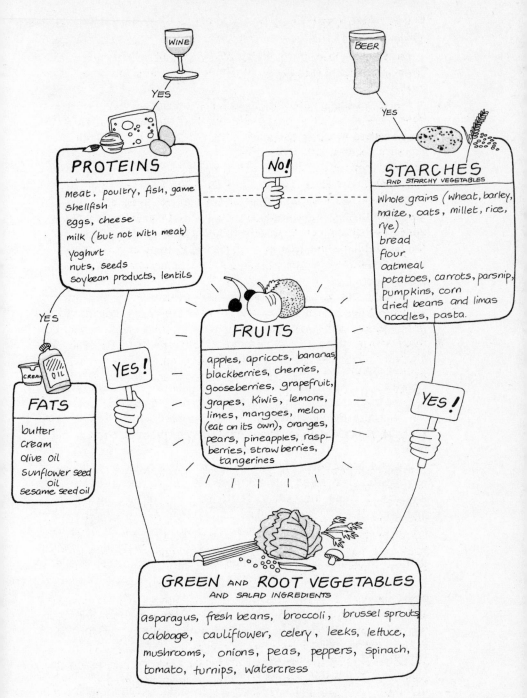

WINE
YES

BEER
YES

PROTEINS

meat, poultry, fish, game
shellfish
eggs, cheese
milk (but not with meat)
yoghurt
nuts, seeds
soybean products, lentils

No!

STARCHES
AND STARCHY VEGETABLES

Whole grains (wheat, barley,
maize, oats, millet, rice,
rye)
bread
flour
oatmeal
potatoes, carrots, parsnip,
pumpkins, corn
dried beans and limas
noodles, pasta.

YES

YES!

FRUITS

apples, apricots, bananas,
blackberries, cherries,
gooseberries, grapefruit,
grapes, kiwis, lemons,
limes, mangoes, melon
(eat on its own), oranges,
pears, pineapples, rasp-
berries, strawberries,
tangerines

YES!

FATS

butter
cream
olive oil
sunflower seed
oil
sesame seed oil

GREEN AND ROOT VEGETABLES
AND SALAD INGREDIENTS

asparagus, fresh beans, broccoli, brussel sprouts,
cabbage, cauliflower, celery, leeks, lettuce,
mushrooms, onions, peas, peppers, spinach,
tomato, turnips, watercress

in *The Dark Side of the Brain* by Harry Oldfield and Roger Coghill. (Element Books, 1988).

1. Cooking in a wok
2. Steaming (as in dim sum)
3. Microwave cooking
4. Pressure cooking and prolonged boiling
5. Deep frying
6. Oven baking

Here is another list of food preservation methods, in the same order – best first.

1. Fresh is best of course – that is, no preservation. Heading the list are freshly caught fish, freshly killed meat and raw food. (This food, cooled in the refrigerator for four hours, is acceptable.) But remember that no food at the butcher's or fishmonger's is really freshly killed or caught, it is a day or two old at least
2. Accelerated freeze-dried
3. Frozen in the ice compartment
4. Gamma irradiated
5. Chemically preserved

Methods 4 and 5 have the worst effect on food.

In killing the bacteria, viruses and fungi that make food 'go off', the chemicals used in method 5 will kill all the life present in the food cells as well. Irradiated food (method 4) is even more dangerous but incredibly (because manufacturers anticipate big profits from the increased shelf-life of foods) it is permitted in the USA and is about to be permitted in Britain.

Gamma irradiation (which is akin to nuclear radiation) kills some food-poisoning bacteria but only disables others, and it leaves other food contaminants unscathed. The ones it kills off are the very ones that warn us – by smell, colour change and so on – that food is off. Irradiation also destroys vitamins and enzymes, prevents fruit from ripening and damages the flesh of food so badly that it is too unripe to eat one day and too bad to eat the next, because after a few days other bacteria take over where the irradiated ones have been temporarily disabled.

No wonder this is being described as the age for taking our health into our own hands. When the nation's food laws do not protect us from situations such as the one described above, it is no wonder that we have to take precautions ourselves.

Looking at our modern, more sedentary lifestyles, our depleted, less nutritious foods and our increasing pollution, there can be little doubt that we need to eat less because we exercise less, but we also need to get more nutrition from our food, because that will protect us from pollution. What's the solution? Try the following.

VITAMIN/MINERAL SUPPLEMENTS: VITAL SPARE PARTS OR FLASHY ACCESSORIES?

To supplement or not to supplement, that is the question most often asked nowadays. And if the answer is yes, what supplement to choose? The plethora of products on the market makes just the job of choosing a supplement a stress risk!

People just don't know, yet they have more to say about supplements than any other issue in the alternative health spectrum. This is especially true of doctors who rarely believe in taking them (which is interesting considering that their nutritional training in medical school is negligible). In this instance they are not talking from knowledge.

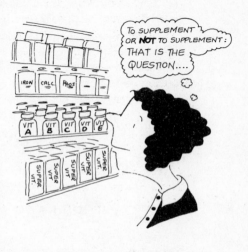

Patrick Holford is (see useful addresses). He is one of the best-known nutritional experts in Britain, but even he admits that this is a difficult area. He points out that every year the British public spend in excess of £100 million on vitamin and mineral supplements, but in his opinion an estimated 60 per cent of the active ingredients literally go down the drain. As he explains, not knowing which form of a nutrient to take, when to take it, and with what, can vitally influence its effectiveness. Also, many VOPs don't realize that vitamins need to be taken together, as their combined effects enhance each other. Some substances aid the uptake of vitamins and minerals into the bloodstream; others, which may be quite common in our diet, block them. He believes that everyone should have expert nutritional advice.

VITAMIN-BLOCKERS

We have all heard of beta-blockers, which block certain nervous reactions, but there are vitamin-blockers too, and their action is not beneficial to the body.

One of the worst culprits in this respect is tea, which blocks the body's absorption of iron by about two-thirds. Coffee is nearly as bad.

Yet how many people take their vitamin pill in the morning with a cup of tea or coffee? Some drinks, such as fresh orange juice, aid the uptake of vitamins. Others, such as alcohol, almost completely negate it. It is really depressing when you realize how much you have to know in order to benefit from vitamins and minerals. This is why Patrick Holford has produced a vitamin-combining chart to show what helps, what hinders and what should be taken with what in the way of supplements. This is reproduced here, and although it is not a complete guide, it will help to minimize the number of errors you make.

THE NUTS AND BOLTS OF NUTRITION

Let's get a few terms straight first. Diet is what you eat; nutrition is what you get out of what you eat. Remember that the word 'diet' does not just mean 'slimming diet'; it refers to your overall eating pattern – what kind of food you normally eat and in what quantity.

Nutrition and understanding how supplements work is a very new science. Body chemistry is so complex that it is only in recent times that we have had any comprehension of what goes on where it all counts – that is, at cellular level – and what we are learning serves only to show how miraculous the human body is, and how worthy of our respect – equally worthy, surely, of a conscientious maintenance programme.

THE FOUR PILLARS OF NUTRITION

VITAMINS
Vitamins are the spark plugs of the body. They are biochemical sub-stances, which can be destroyed by heat, which means that any but the lightest of cooking puts paid to them rapidly (refer to Harry Oldfield's list of cooking techniques given earlier in this chapter).

The body uses vitamins to make all the quantities of enzymes that it needs for its thousand and one chemical reactions. Enzymes are also the body's first line of defence – they are present in the lining of the lungs and in the lining of the stomach, and they come into play far sooner than the better known immune system response of the white corpuscles. So if a vitamin is missing, a vital enzyme may be deficient, and may drag our defences down as a result.

Most nutritional experts (as opposed to doctors) think that we need to take a vitamin supplement every day of our lives. Because vitamins work in conjunction with the second pillar of nutrition, minerals, it is advisable to take them together in what is called a multi-vitamin and mineral supplement. Everyone knows that in an ideal world we wouldn't have to take them, but few would argue that we are living in an ideal world.

Children also need a vitamin-mineral supplement. Trials on both sides of the Atlantic have shown how such supplements can favourably affect children's I.Q., as well as resistance to common childhood complaints. Behaviour is favourably affected too (see Chapter 7).

MINERALS

Minerals are more stable than vitamins, fortunately, which might lead the average reader to believe that they are in relatively good supply in the body. Not so. Although they can't be destroyed like vitamins, they can be lost, either by too-rigorous food processing (chromium is lost this way) or because the soil from which minerals are derived, is itself depleted and polluted (selenium is lost because of this). Both chromium and selenium are vital trace minerals, which protect the body from the effects of ageing, and indications show that we are not getting enough of these from a normal, daily diet.

Factors such as this offer the only rebuttal needed to those who say

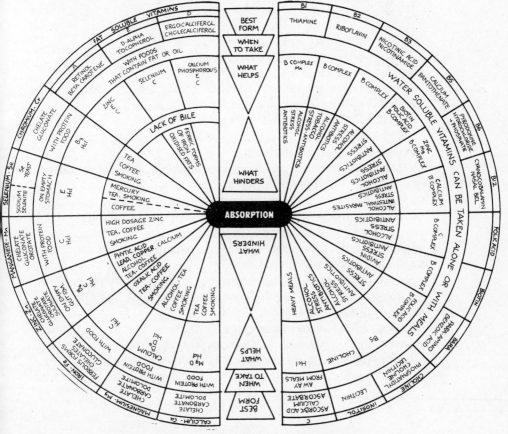

Supplied Courtesy of the Institute for Optimum Nutrition

we do not need supplements if we have a wholesome diet. Perhaps with a lot of care and by reverting to organic farming and careful food processing, we will be able to say so again – *in time*.

Minerals are the building blocks of the body: for example, calcium is needed to make strong bones and teeth. They, like vitamins, form a vital part of the body's defence system in much the same way that treatment for rust preserves a car chassis.

Shortly, we will get to the nuts and bolts of what to take. Some people might call those nuts and bolts the RDAs (Recommended Daily Allowance levels). We will have nothing to do with those, since they are a bit like social security payments, calculated to keep you alive, not much more.

AMINO ACIDS AND PERSONAL NUTRITIONAL REQUIREMENTS

These bear no relationship to the rather more sinister kinds of acid, which are becoming all-too-popular these days.

Amino acids are the building blocks of the body, and they are derived mainly from the proteins we consume. (Proteins are a vital part of our diet, as are carbohydrates and fats.) Everyone must have some protein intake to live, even, and especially, vegetarians and vegans, who must take their protein from vegetable sources such as nuts, grains, and pulses, and if they do not replace the protein they would normally have had from animal sources, they may become very sick indeed.

Strictly speaking, if we eat a balanced diet of proteins, fats and carbohydrates we should not need to supplement it with amino acids. Their use should be considered only if an annoying condition or symptom persists in spite of vitamin supplementation. Amino acids are occasionally needed by inexperienced vegetarians or vegans who are not getting enough protein in their specialized diets. At this level you should seek advice from a nutritional expert.

The above-mentioned nutritional nuts and bolts, down to the last tiny screw, must be present in order to make a sound and healthy body able to withstand the slings and arrows of life. It should be possible to produce a formula which covers the average nutritional requirement, but, as if to throw another spanner in the works, modern nutritional experts have discovered that we all have different requirements due to differences in build, lifestyle, diet, ease of absorption and so on. There is no such thing as an average human being when it comes to nutrition.

Dosage cannot be suggested for the above reasons, but safe indications are usually given on the labels.

A top quality multi-vitamin/mineral supplement every day should be your basic survival kit. In addition, you may consider taking extra vitamin A (in the safe form of Beta Carotene), vitamin E (in the pure form of D-Alpha Tocopherol) and natural vitamin C (with bioflavonoids) because these three vitamins protect the body from ageing. Essential fatty acids, taken in the form of cod liver oil or EPA capsules, protect blood vessels and keep cholesterol levels in check, while evening primrose complements their effect as well as helping some forms of PMT.

Vitamins should be taken with food in the mornings; minerals should be taken at night – but they can be taken together. Keep all oil-based vitamins in the refrigerator to stop them becoming rancid. It is important not to take vitamin A in the form of Retinol and vitamin D in excess. Do not exceed the levels and dosages contained in your multi-vitamin supplement unless you are advised to do so by a qualified practitioner.

SPECIAL SUBSTANCES: ADAPTOGENS

Everyone has heard of ginseng, royal jelly (which should be taken fresh) and more recently of lapacho, the Brazilian rain-forest herb. (See Useful Addresses under Rio Trading.) These products are known as adaptogens, which simply means that their beneficial effects on the body adapt to its specific needs. Nobody really knows how they work, but a short course of one or other of them when you are feeling jaded can often work wonders. Pfaffia, another Brazilian herb, is used to alleviate menopausal conditions. Catuba is to men what Pfaffia is to women.

Adaptogens should not be taken all the time, but simply to help recovery from an illness or from stress and fatigue, say, a month's course a year. Chlorella, spirulina and green-lipped mussels are also useful under certain circumstances. All these possibilities point to:

GETTING NUTRITIONAL ADVICE!

Before offering you any more advice, here is some good news for those who feel totally overwhelmed and bewildered by the myriad of avenues of therapeutic, nutritional and options that are mentioned here. In nearly every major town and city alternative health practices have sprung up in the last few years. Nearly every major nutritional supplier has a nutritional advisor available for free advice. Some health food stores have a consultant available at weekends.

Due care and caution are advised: like everyone else, people working in alternative and nutritional health want to make money, but most of them do care – they have often started up on a shoestring because of their beliefs. With sifting and awareness, you can usually find exactly the advice and help you may need. Finally, a good guideline to follow is to realize that you get what you pay for: more expensive vitamins are not a 'con': it means that the ingredients used are more bio-available – you will actually get to absorb what you are taking.

EMPHASIZING ELIMINATION

For a long time now, it was thought that if we ate a good diet we would be well-protected from the ailments of life. 'Eat up or you'll get sick' was a favourite phrase of our parents, and nobody was allowed to get down from the table having left any food – which was usually well and truly cooked, by the way. Soggy, even. Now we know that we in the West have been digging our graves with our teeth. The average American is overweight and has been described by key American medical figure Dr Dwight McKee as having 70 billion 'garbage cans' for cells. The average Briton, if not overweight, is usually in a perpetual battle against the bulge.

The irony of the situation is that the bodies of people who live in so-called deprived and undernourished areas of the world are far less toxic than those of Westerners. Of course, there comes a point when undernourishment does its own damage, but the fact remains that we have been concentrating far too much on digestion and far too little on evacuation. That so many people in the West are overweight is as much due to absorption of pollutants, which require fat to be stored in the body to accommodate them, as from overeating.

Implausible? Think about it. Ask your grandmother to recall the days when people used to have a 'cuppa' with bread and butter or a biscuit first thing in the morning, followed by a hearty breakfast, then cake or biscuits at elevenses, followed by a cooked lunch, afternoon tea of cucumber sandwiches followed by tea or dinner (depending on which term you prefer), and finally supper, a nice mug of milky drink plus a bedtime snack ... not forgetting the odd sweet or box of chocolates consumed between. Never have we eaten so little and, by comparison, put on so much weight!

Pollution provides the grim clue. There are indications that in the latter half of the 20th century we are being exposed to unprecedented levels of industrial waste and the results of untold quantities of chemicals being poured onto our crops and farmlands every year, and they are finding their way not only into our food but into the Earth's water supply and we are drinking (and breathing) a concoction of chemicals every day. The liver, struggling to cope with such chemical overload, is making fat deposits in which to store it, just as deposits to store nuclear and other wastes are being constructed every day for similar reasons. We are fat because fat is saving our lives!

Of course, there will always be thin people and people whose strong livers manage to keep up with today's toxic cocktail of chemicals, but the average person is not keeping up with their toxic load, and we need to do extra things now that we didn't need to do before.

THE TEN GOLDEN RULES OF ELIMINATION

1. Drink plenty of pure water, and eat foods that have a high water content. Water is a wonderful solvent and flusher-out of toxins, not only for the kidneys and bladder, but for the colon too.
2. Go on a weekend fruit fast. Consume as much fresh fruit and drink as much pure fruit juice as you want, but be sure to eat only fruit for two days. On the Friday evening beforehand, have a light meal of steamed or grilled fish, or better still have a vegetarian meal. On the Monday after your diet, get back slowly to eating other foods. Ease your way in, otherwise you will have undone much of the good. This diet should be tried on a quiet weekend when you are able to rest.
3. Get to grips with constipation. This is an insidious condition, which results in your re-absorbing your own toxins. A daily ration of oat bran will tone up the colon and, for good measure, the blood vessels. Eat plenty of fresh fruit and vegetables – not frozen – such as cabbage, beans and root vegetables, but not too many potatoes. If you have to resort to laxatives, take a spoonful of psyllium husks or linseeds in a good-sized glass of fresh fruit juice. Both are available in health food stores. Remember that regular laxatives leach out valuable minerals.
4. Cut down on all drug-taking, even aspirin. Drugs are chemicals. Keep a little pot of feverfew on your windowsill and chew a few leaves if you have a headache.
5. Take acidophilus to keep the intestinal flora balanced, since they too deal with toxins.
6. Limit your drinking and smoking and take plenty of vitamin C (see Nutrition), which hastens food along the gut and combats the effects of drinking and smoking.
7. Don't eat much before midday – this gives the liver a fighting chance.
8. Buy a colon cleanse pack from one of the reputable health suppliers (see Useful Addresses) and use it every six months or better still (easier and more effective) have a course of colonic irrigation once a year to cleanse the colon. When performed by a properly trained practitioner – and there are more and more of them being

trained – this treatment is as good for you as a de-coke is for an old car full of carbon deposits and is completely harmless. This is not an unpleasant treatment, in fact quite the reverse. Purified water is gently introduced into the colon, where it flushes out, layer by layer, all the deposits adhering to the colon walls, thus inhibiting their muscular expulsion/evacuation movements. There are differing schools of colonic therapeutic practice, but I recommend choosing a therapist who uses disposable insertion junctions and who gives an implant of acidophilus afterwards.

After a course of colonic irrigation, many people notice that their skin colour is a healthier hue, that they have lost weight and generally feel lighter. It is a very good way of controlling candida overgrowth as well. People still think of this as a kinky therapy, but this is because we are so screwed up about that part of the body. This has to change! Test yourself by answering this question: What is the difference between having tubes inserted into your blood vessels, as the medical profession is wont to do under all sorts of circumstances, and having tubes inserted into a natural opening?
9. Test food sensitivities you suspect you may have by kinesology or dowsing (see chapter 12) and eliminate!
10. Read chapter 10 and learn to use other ways to prompt elimination besides the colon.

DIET EXAMINATION TIME
Finally, if you have stayed the pace through this mammoth chapter, are you ready to look back on the list of foods you owned up to in your typical diet and give yourself a mark out of 10? When I look back on the years that my score would have been nought or one or two out of 10, I marvel at how forgiving my body has been to me.

5

*

THE HEART AND CIRCULATORY SYSTEM

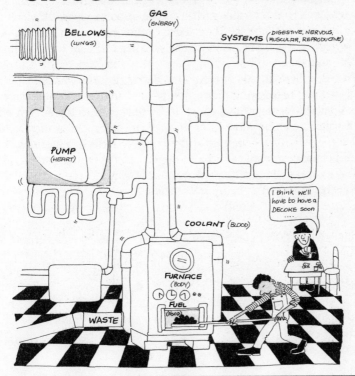

IN THIS CHAPTER

* System workings * Heartbeat factors * Blood and blood pressure * Coronary care * Varicose veins * How arteries get clogged * The de-clog process * Cholesterol: friend or foe? * Sussing your circulatory symptoms * Heart-felt nutrition * Chelation therapy: new way to bypass bypass * Self-help for stress and hyperventilation * Road-checking your circulatory system

Coronary heart disease (CHD) was virtually unheard of at the beginning of this century. Now Britain has the highest level of CHD of all the developed countries, with most English-speaking countries following closely behind. Virtually everyone is at risk from CHD and other disorders of the circulatory system, which, together with cancer, are two of our greatest contemporary killers. Both are degenerative diseases – that is, diseases brought about by the body's inability to keep up with the daily repair work necessary to service the system.

Unfortunately transport systems, bringing as they do the life blood to the entity they serve, are very unforgiving of neglect. Sewerage systems can go neglected for years, as is the case in many cities, of which London is a prime example. They cause problems eventually, but not initially, just as the body's elimination systems will take years of neglect before they finally rebel.

However, imagine what would happen if London Transport stopped servicing its buses, or London Underground its trains. It takes only one signal failure for much of London to be disrupted as the system grinds to a halt. The same must be true of every major city of the world. In the same way, the failure of a tiny coronary artery, measuring a few centimetres long, can lead to an untimely and even permanent disruption – possibly the death of the system.

Yet the body's circulatory system is little short of miraculous, consisting as it does of a double, self-priming, self-servicing pump that even the cleverest engineers have been unable to duplicate, plus at least 96,000km (60,000 miles) (estimates vary) of tough, elasticized, self-repairing, heavy-duty piping called blood vessels, through which flows about 5 litres (9 pints) of a miraculous living substance, really a tissue in itself but also a transportation, repair, refuse-removing, germ-fighting, temperature-maintaining and re-generating liquid called blood. And, all this is tucked tidily into the 'five-feet-something' framework of the human body.

THE HEART

The focal point, the driving force, of the system is, of course, the heart, which is positioned centrally in the body behind the sternum or breast bone, with its lower chambers angled slightly to the left. It is the size of a clenched fist, but in that pocket-sized organ are two strong pumps which work quite separately from each other, though not independently.

The heart's job is closely tied up with the lungs and breathing, because one of its main functions is to pump oxygenized blood from the lungs to every bit of body tissue, and then to return it to the lungs for the elimination of carbon dioxide followed by re-oxygenization. Of course in the process other vital supplies are transported around the body as well, such as nutrients from the digestive system, enzymes and hormones from the glandular system, as well as waste products from the body's main chemical process, oxidative phosphorylation, whereby energy for life is generated. (Remember, the body is really a furnace in which controlled burning takes place at discreet temperatures in order to produce energy for life.)

Naturally, the smooth running of all of this activity depends on the efficiency of the pump driving the liquid coolant (blood) around the furnace, the viscosity of the coolant, the state of the pipes and the efficient removal of the waste products of burning (including the gases). If all or any one of these processes malfunctions, then the circulation suffers.

The heart pumps blood round the tissues at the incredible rate of 5 litres (9 pints) a minute. To do this it pumps continuously from a few weeks after the fertilization of the egg, while it is still in the womb, until death. Calculating lifespan as averaging 75 years this represents a stunning performance of $72 \times 60 \times 24 \times 365.25 \times 75$ = approximately 3,000,000,000 beats, or 40 million beats a year.

The left side of the heart is the larger of the pumps – in fact, all the other bits of the heart wrap themselves around it. This pumps bright red oxygenated blood to the body systems, which for this reason is called systemic circulation. The right side of the heart pumps the dark, carbon dioxide-containing blood to the lungs for its elimination and reoxygenation, which is called pulmonary circulation. For a fuller description of this process see Chapter 6.

A LOOK INSIDE THE HEART

The heart has four chambers, two at each side. The two upper ones have thin muscular walls and are called atria (think of atrium, meaning receiving chamber). These receive the blood from the main veins bearing blood to the heart and pass it through to two much thicker walled, larger, lower chambers called ventricles, which pump the blood through the arteries to the rest of the body. This is done by squeezing the blood onwards, so the walls need to be very tough but elastic. The cardiac muscle tissue which constitutes the walls is unique in the body.

Between the large blood vessels which lead to and from the heart are valves, and between the atria and ventricles are still more valves. These allow blood to flow in only one direction. Most people will have heard of mitral valves and tricuspid valves (and possibly of semilunar valves) because surgeons replace them when they go wrong.

HEART SOUNDS

The opening of the valves is silent, but their closure is what gives the heart its characteristic sounds. As blood is propelled first through the atrial valves and then, a fraction of a second later, through the ventrical valves, two sounds, phonetically 'lubb' and 'dup', occur, the first when the atrial valves close, the second when the valves between the ventricles and the main arteries close (to stop backflow of blood into the heart).

After this exertion these is a tiny pause while the heart rests before it goes on. So we hear: 'lubb-dup', pause, 'lubb-dup', pause.

ELECTROCARDIOGRAPHS

An electrocardiograph depicts and records this rythm in graph form, giving the familiar normal heart-beat pattern often displayed during popular TV programmes with a health theme. Any disorder affecting the electrical impulses and their conduction through the heart or on cardiac muscle response shows on the EEG, which is why it is now preferred for diagnostic purposes instead of just listening to the sounds the heart makes through a stethoscope, although even that can be informative. Heart murmurs, for example, when valves dysfunction, are clearly heard, sometimes even without a stethoscope.

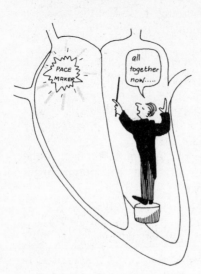

ORIGIN OF THE HEARTBEAT

This is one of the wonders of life. What makes the rudimentary foetal heart start beating? That it does so long before the rudimentary nervous system begins to function is even more astonishing. Several factors are at work. The first is that cardiac muscle contracts rythmically of its own accord, right from its inception. If a bit of it is taken from a heart and put in a culture in a laboratory, it goes on contracting. So it doesn't require any messages from the nervous system to do this – unlike all other muscles, which are dependent on the electrical impulses carried to them through the nerves from the brain.

Second, the heart has a natural pacemaker, which is also independent of the central nervous system (CNS). This directs and orchestrates the heartbeat from its position in the right atrium of the heart. This node has the ability to generate an electric (action) potential which spreads, via a second node in the right ventricle, through the heart. This it does 72 times a minute, which is why it is called a pacemaker.

Thus the heart's natural impulse is to beat 72 times a minute.

In real life this is modified by other factors – that is, it is speeded or slowed by additional input from the CNS. Regrettably for mankind this system (see Chapter 7) is affected by stress, so that stressors can have a direct result on heartbeat rate, usually increasing it. Left to its own devices, the heart would beat quite regularly without this, but the interference has to be there, or we would not be able to call on the heart to respond to our needs, e.g. to work faster when we want to run or to slow down when we want to rest.

MIGHTY MINERALS AND ARTERIAL PLAQUES

There is a third important factor affecting heartbeat, which is that the electrical (action) potential is generated by a delicate balance in the concentrations of sodium, potassium and calcium, groups of atoms of which carry the positive or negative charges needed to generate the body electricity. Obviously we can interfere directly with heart function, depressing it, for example, if we over-eat salt (see Chapter 7), as our modern diet tends to encourage, and under-eat fresh fruit in which potassium is found.

Calcium is another double-edged sword in the cardiac equation. The heart is so sensitive to the right calcium balance that before it is disturbed, calcium will be precipitated out of the bloodstream into the tissues. Unfortunately, some of it gets laid down in the arterial walls as a complement to excess cholesterol, making hard, plaque-like deposits, which narrow these vessels, causing the heart to have to work harder to pump blood through them.

An added threat is that bits of this calcium deposit, just like lime in pipes, tend to break off into the bloodstream and can be carried along until they reach smaller blood vessels, such as in the coronary arteries or even in the brain, where they can block circulation, causing heart attacks or strokes. Tissue must have its blood supply to live and function, otherwise it wastes away and dies.

Obviously we need calcium, but from middle-age onwards we do not need as much as we did when we were young. Yet still our diet induces us to overeat it, in the form of much favoured dairy products – milk, cream, cheese, yoghurt, butter – and in the form of seeds, nuts and cereals.

The body will do a fine job of coping with our dietary vicissitudes but it is not infallible, as recent coronary heart disease figures show. We must do our bit by eating the right diet, and as we get older there is less and less room for error.

BLOOD PRESSURE

The action of the heartbeat (actually a wringing motion which drives the blood onwards) generates blood pressure.

Each ventricle, at each heartbeat, propels about 70ml (0.14 pint) of blood into the blood vessels. Although the blood vessels are extremely elastic, this is nonetheless a big influx of blood for them to handle, and they do so in two stages. Nearly half the blood moves with the heart beat, but the other half is held in the expanded tissues and moved forwards while the heart is resting between beats. This accounts for pressure being at its highest at the height of the heart's contraction (that is, systolic BP) and at its lowest when the heart is relaxing (that is, diastolic BP). The average for these two figures is 120/80. The difference between the two figures is important because it tells the doctor how elastic the blood vessels are or aren't – that is, what resistance the heart is meeting from the blood vessels when it requires them to expand to take the full consignment of blood pumped. Obviously, if they are narrowed by cholesterol and calcium deposits, or simply by tension, diastolic pressure will remain high and the heart will have to work against this resistance. All the more reason, therefore, to try to keep the blood vessels clear to avoid straining both the pump and the pipes.

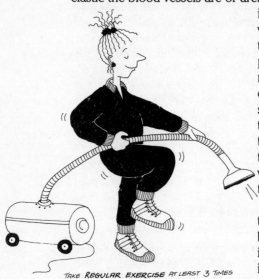

TAKE REGULAR EXERCISE AT LEAST 3 TIMES A WEEK .....

Blood pressure is also affected by the chemical composition of the blood; if it is thicker than it should be it is more difficult, e.g. too much fat in the blood makes it thicker.

A decreased oxygen or increased carbon dioxide tension also causes a reflex elevation of blood pressure. Respiratory activity is, therefore, an important regulator of arterial pressure. Naturally it would have to be: if we start exerting ourselves we must breathe faster because we need to get more oxygen to the muscles we are using. The heart must then beat faster to transport that oxygen to the muscle groups we are exerting; in other words, there is a feed-back system at work between the heart and lungs.

BLOOD PRESSURE AND EXERCISE

Aerobic exercise to keep this feed-back system in good functioning order is beneficial to the heart and lungs, since it makes the blood move faster, bringing much needed oxygen and nutrients to the tissues and flushing out the debris (wastes) of the body's chemical processes. Our sedentary lifestyles – note that word again, linked to sediment and ageing (see

Chapter 3) – are responsible for a doubling in the risk of heart disease. However, it is important that aerobic exercise is taken on a regular basis (at least three times per week, preferably for 15 minutes a time), otherwise the heart may be strained by sudden, too vigorous activity.

Choose from the following: jogging (but read about its drawbacks in Chapter 8), swimming, skipping, using a mini-rebounder, brisk walking (for half an hour) or even vigorous household activities such as vacuuming and bed-making!

Just as it is important to keep other muscles in working order, it is even more vital to keep the heart muscle in trim.

TEST YOUR HEART FITNESS

To test whether your heart is resilient and able to respond to your needs, exercise for 10 minutes, rest for exactly one minute, and then take your pulse for 30 seconds and double the count. It should be about 100 at this point. If it is more than 130, you are out of condition or your exercise was far too strenuous. Remember this golden rule: exercise does not ensure that your heart is in good condition but lack of it is a risk factor.

THE VITAL VULNERABLE CORONARY ARTERIES

Because the heart is a sealed watertight pump, it cannot depend for oxygen and nourishment on the blood contained in its chambers. Also, when muscles work, they give off waste products, and these have to be taken away like any factory waste. Thus, the heart has to have its own blood supply, and it gets this from two coronary arteries, which branch off the aorta, or main artery, and curl back round the heart for this purpose, sending out a network of 'twigs' through the muscular walls. The fact that they are end arteries and have few cross-connections and that they are little (about the size of matchsticks) means that they have a tendency to get blocked, and when they do, the part of the heart muscle they are serving goes out of action. This is a frequent cause of myocardial infarct or heart attack.

If the part of the heart suffering from muscle starvation happens to involve one of the nodes or pacemakers, obviously that is cause for an artificial pacemaker to be fitted.

All these life-and-death crises require the emergency measures of interventive medicine, but how much better to practise preventive measures achieved by diet and by learning breathing and relaxation techniques.

HEART PAIN
It is an interesting fact that heart pain is not actually felt in the heart itself, so warnings may be disguised. This is because there are no nerves within the heart itself, hence pain is not felt on site but often in the neck or left arm – what is known as referred pain.

THE CIRCULATION OF THE BLOOD

Blood from the body enters the right-hand side of the heart through the main veins or venae cavae. It then passes from the right atrium to the right ventricle, which pumps it to the lungs through the pulmonary arteries.

There it gives off its carbon dioxide and takes on a new consignment of oxygen, in the process changing from bluish-red to bright orangey-red. It then arrives back to the heart and through the pulmonary vein, enters the left-hand side of the heart, passes through the left atrium to the left ventricle, from where it will be pumped (this time under great pressure as it has to go a long way) through the aorta to the organs and extremities.

BODY SYSTEMS CIRCULATION
This is achieved through a closed system of tubes that, together with the heart, function very much like a central heating system. For the successful transportation of blood it is of paramount importance that the tubes (arteries) are not furred up and that they retain their elasticity, because of course the fact that they do not, due to modern diet and lifestyle, means that arterial deterioration is responsible for at least 40 per cent of all deaths in the Western world. But it is controllable, once what is happening is known. As famous health writer Gayelord Hauser once said: 'health can be re-built at any age.'

From the arteries the blood goes to progressively tinier arteries (arterioles). The arterioles lead into millions (about 10 billion actually) of even more minute capillaries, the walls of which are only one cell in thickness and which act as semi-permeable membranes. It is in this network that oxygen and nutrients are drawn off by body tissues and exchanged for the waste products of cell metabolism, including carbon dioxide.

As the capillaries converge on the other side of their leaf-like networks, small veins (venules) begin to collect the blood and re-direct it back to the heart. Because by this stage there is very little blood pressure, valves similar to those in the heart, allowing the blood to flow in only one direction, propel the blood towards the larger veins and eventually to the vena cava, which leads into the heart.

Veins have much thinner walls than arteries because they do not need to withstand such pressures.

VARICOSE VEINS

When the valves fail to do their job successfully in directing the blood towards the heart, vein engorgement occurs, and this disposes the veins to increase in girth. These become varicose veins, a condition that tends to run in families, some members of whom escape, some don't.

There are two types of varicose veins – those on the surface, which are unsightly but give less trouble, and those that are deep, which are more painful. Since exercising the leg muscles helps the veins to contract and the valves to work better, walking is one of the best solutions to this problem. Standing in one spot is, of course, fatal, yet it is one of life's little ironies that people who suffer from this complaint often work as cooks, shop assistants or schoolteachers.

Constipation should be avoided since it adds to internal downward pressure, whether the veins are in the legs or, as in the case of the other common type of varicose veins (haemorrhoids), in the rectum.

HAEMORRHOIDS

It has been said: cure constipation (see Chapter 4) and you will cure haemorrhoids, and this is almost invariably true. However, the way to approach this problem is not by taking laxatives, but by introducing natural fibre into the diet in the form of fresh fruit, vegetables, oat bran (rather than wheat bran which leaches valuable minerals from the body) and by drinking plenty of pure, bottled water. (Oat bran also helps to control cholesterol levels.)

Witch hazel suppositories work very well for haemorrhoids, as do other herbal remedies for varicose veins of the legs. A visit to a knowledgeable herbalist should always be attempted before resorting to an operation. If veins are taken away, greater strain is put on the ones remaining.

Changes in diet are also recommended, with the avoidance of all smoked and pickled foods. Alcohol, chocolate and rhubarb also seem to aggravate veins in this condition, although trial and error will tell most people what they can and cannot eat.

ARTERIES AND THEIR CONSTRUCTION

The walls of arteries differ from the thinner walled veins because they need to convey blood under pressure. Actually they are a bit like good quality garden hoses, complete with the rose system to cut down pressure if needed. There is an internal surface which is very smooth to facilitate blood flow, an elasticized muscular layer, which contracts or relaxes with the pulse, and a tougher, more fibrous but elastic outer layer, to withstand the high pressures within.

When arteries are healthy they function like bouncy rubber; when they are not they are rather like rubber that has been left out in the sun. It is obvious that when arteries reach that condition they will not successfully cope with the huge daily throughput of blood required of them. In fact each drop of blood in our bodies probably travels further than most people walk per day – 3 kilometres ($1\frac{3}{4}$ miles).

A BRIEF WORD ABOUT BLOOD

Anyone who has not seen living blood through a microscope, preferably their own living blood, has missed one of the Attenborough-style wonders of life. Under one's very gaze it can be seen to be full of a variety of particles, some actively moving about while carrying out their tasks of digesting foreign substances or organizing themselves into certain areas, etc., others moving purposefully forward as if directed by a drill sergeant. An army of several divisions seems to be on the march, carrying supplies, clearing debris and getting rid of enemy forces.

In fact, the blood does contain a variety of cells, which are replaced about every four months from new ones made mainly in the bone marrow or lymph glands. Some cells (erythrocytes) carry oxygen, others (leukocytes of many types) are part of the immune system and are there for our protection (see Chapter 11). Their job is to digest foreign bacteria or to combine with them in such a way as to put them out of action.

There are also platelets, the coagulating agents that come into force if we cut ourselves so that we do not bleed to death. Haemophilia is a condition in which this blood function does not work, and the affected person is likely to bleed to death from a relatively small cut.

The viscosity of the blood – in facts its entire composition – is a sure indicator of health or otherwise, which is why blood tests are the most common of all health tests. The blood comes in contact with every part of the body and its contents tell the story of what is or is not going on.

CHOLESTEROL! FRIEND OR FOE?

Believe it or not, cholesterol is a vital part of the blood. We have come to believe that it is the enemy of life, but it is only in excess that it is undesirable. It is an oily, slippery substance, not water soluble, so it is suspended in globules in the blood for transportation, and is a vital component of nerve transmission, hormones, cell membranes and of the digestive substance, bile. Cholesterol is actually manufactured in the body, as well as produced from the foods we eat. In order to be carried around it is bound to a protein called lipoprotein, a low-density protein known as LDL. If there is too much cholesterol circulating, the body re-binds it to a high-density protein (HDL) and returns it to the liver to be excreted through the bile.

The problem with modern diets is that they tend to provide us with more LDL than HDL, thus disposing of the cholesterol is made more difficult. This fact was discovered by studying Eskimos, who, despite their huge intake of fats, rarely seemed to get heart disease. The significant factor was discovered to be in the type of fats they ate. These were largely fish oils, very rich in HDLs. For this reason many heart specialists now recommend that their patients take EFAs (essential fatty acids) such as cod liver oil or halibut oil, or eat oily fish at least once a week. (All oils or oil supplements must be refrigerated or they go rancid – an even worse factor for the body to deal with). A good oil to take in supplement form is EPA (eicosapentaenoic acid), not to be confused with EFA, which simply means essential fatty acid.

THE FAT FACTOR IN HEART DISEASE

Cholesterol has got a very bad name, not altogether deserved, as it is only one of the rogues in the heart disease equation. The problem is that the average Western diet contains no less than 40 per cent fat, most of which is hidden from view so that it is not realised that they are being eaten, such as in sausages, hamburgers, salamis and in cold, frozen and tinned meat and fish, as well as in biscuits, pastries, sweets and even in ice-cream.

The reasons for their inclusion are:
1. Fat is cheap.
2. Fat is tasty, as anyone knows who has ever savoured the skin of roast chicken or the crackling of pork.

To make matters worse, what isn't hidden and consumed in tinned, processed and frozen foods as fat is often hidden and consumed as sugar, which is converted into yet more fat because that is how the body stores and transports its excess stores of food. Sugar is included in nearly every product to make it tastier, even in soups, pasta sauces and liquids such as tomato juice.

Anyone wanting to know just how bad processed sugar is for the human body should read *Pure, White and Deadly* by John Yudkin.

What does the body do with this fatty plenitude? In order to get it out of the bloodstream, where too much would have a clogging effect as surely as pouring a dish of fat down a sink, it deposits it on the walls of the nearest object, the arteries. But this is not all; the picture is further complicated by other misguided dietary habits. Turning for a moment from cholesterol, it is useful to look at the whole picture of the causes of arterial disease, a disease which kills 200,000 men and women in the UK each year (and similar proportions of people in other Western Countries), many of them long before their three-score years and ten.

WHAT IS HEART DISEASE?

Heart disease is in fact arterial disease, so it is wrongly named. When people hear that so and so has died of a heart attack, what is meant in most cases is that the arteries feeding the heart muscle became blocked, causing heart failure. Strokes are just another example of arterial disease: this time the blockage is in the brain. Intermittent claudication, pain on walking, is yet another example, this time of the arteries leading to the legs.

The process of arterial disease is years long, and unfortunately it is usually quite silent until the artery is 90 or even 95 per cent blocked. Young people happily smoking away or eating masses of hamburgers and chips have no idea of the process they are starting. In fact, when autopsies were carried out on young American casualties of the Vietnam War whose average age was 22, and who were, presumably, very fit, it was discovered that most of them had arterial disease. The American diet is worse, if anything, than the British diet in respect of being a contributory factor, since there even more fast-food is eaten and even more ices, sweets, soft drinks and dairy produce are consumed.

Because of the silent way in which arterial disease begins, many people are unaware of it until it is far advanced. Then they lose hope, thinking that nothing can be done when in fact a great deal can be done.

FIGHT THAT FEAR!
The element of fear also causes a number of people to ignore early symptoms they may have, thinking that by burying their heads in the sand, at least they won't have the worry of knowing they are in danger: i.e. latent rather than blatant fears are preferred. Once again this attitude arises because of the general belief that once you have arterial disease there is nothing to be done about it.

In fact one fairly new therapy, which is described later in this chapter, has a success rate even with advanced sufferers who have had three or four by-pass operations, as well as with those who have been victims of strokes or actual heart attacks, or who are suffering from severe intermittent claudication. However it is obvious that the earlier these conditions are recognized, the better are the chances of recovery.

It is for this reason, and this reason alone, that a list of symptoms has been included that might indicate early problems. If you have several of them, you may be wise to have a check-up, because then and only then can you start on your journey of recovery.

Important: the following symptoms, with the possible exception of angina (heart spasm pain) and high blood pressure are all signs of harmless conditions as well as of less harmless ones. Acknowlege your symptoms by all means, but let an expert diagnose them!

SYMPTOMS OF ARTERIAL DISEASE

● Tingling of the lips

● Frequent headaches or a feeling of heaviness or fullness in the head

● Vision problems

● Feeling terribly emotional, impatient, volatile, pent up

● Buzzing or ringing in the ears (there are many other causes for this)

● Dizziness

● Nose bleeds

● Feeling tired all the time, even in the morning

● Blood pressure that has been diagnosed as too high by a doctor

● Lumps or streaks of fat in the skin close to the eye

● Angina (pain in the chest on exertion or stress)

● Pain in the leg muscles (cramps) on exerting them

● Cold extremities

● Deep, diagonal creases on the lower ear lobe, which may indicate the sort of energy-flow disturbance that is characteristic of coronary problems.

If you suspect that you have arterial disease, awareness of how your lifestyle may have contributed to it is all important, and you may never be told of this by your doctor. For example, it is amazing just how head-in-the-sand the medical profession has been until recently about the overwhelming evidence that diet plays such a huge part in the equation.

CAUSES AND PROCESS OF ARTERIAL DISEASE

There is no doubt that modern dietary habits are a major contributory factor to the increase in arterial disease. However, factors of lifestyle and of what could be called the 20th century also feature. The causes of arterial disease are still being discovered, and the picture is by no means complete. Moreover, what happens is so complex that no one factor can be blamed entirely. Why can one person eat eggs and still have a normal cholesterol level, while another can not? Why can one person smoke without apparent symptoms, while another shows all the signs of circulatory distress? Why can one person lead an incredibly unfit and stressful life and stay well, while another person has a heart attack despite what seems to be a very fit and stable life pattern?

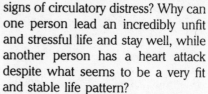

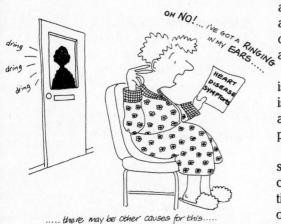

..... *there may be other causes for this* .....

What is happening to the arteries is easier to comprehend than why it is happening. Beginning with the clearer picture, this is an outline of the process.

First, the artery walls get damaged, sometimes by crystals in the blood, called oxides, sometimes by an infection, sometimes by the direct action of free radicals. Free radicals are incomplete oxygen molecules carried in the blood which have an uneven electrical charge. They are the products of pollution and of burning processes such as are released in cigarette and city smoke, car fumes, smoked and barbecued foods, burned fats, etc. Free radicals are like rioters, attacking healthy cells in the most accessible places such as the arterial walls, in order to neutralize their unbalanced charge. In doing so, they damage the cell mechanism, and the cells start to malfunction. Worse, they often start a chain reaction where one robs another of an electron which robs another, so that surrounding cells get damaged too.

When cells get damaged they begin to malfunction. Instead of clearing themselves of toxins and waste products these begin to accumulate in and around them, clinging to the normally smooth arterial walls like bits of flotsam on the uneven sides of a river. Calcium is then attracted to this conglomeration, and the fatty aggregation becomes hardened by it, just as it does in the mouth around bits of food in the teeth. Eventually this plaque sticks out from the walls into the bloodstream, where it attracts other debris.

Ultimately the damaged cells lose their ability to control their growth rate, and they actually begin to proliferate like cancer. They form further bumps of tissue, which stick out into the bloodstream, and this debris completely blocks the smaller arteries. In the case of the larger ones, bits may break off from the plaque-like deposits and get carried along in the bloodstream until they become stuck in smaller arteries, where blood clots may form because the blood becomes stagnant. The words 'thrombosis' and 'embolism' describe situations where clots have formed or been carried along in the bloodstream until they arrive at a passage where they can go no further. If this happens to a vital artery in the heart, lung or brain, a heart attack, pulmonary embolism or stroke can result.

This process is not new: it has always existed to some extent, but it did not seem to affect our forefathers as it now does us because they did not live in industrialized cities surrounded as we are by free-radical producing smoke and car fumes; they did not eat highly processed convenience foods full of yet more free radicals; and they did not lead such stressful lives, jammed up against each other. They also took more natural exercise. Until just over a century and a half ago, most people worked outside, grew their own produce and ate it in natural and simple forms. In fact, their way of life is now providing useful information about how to redress this unhealthy situation.

TURNING BACK THE CLOCK TO CURE CIRCULATORY PROBLEMS
By examining what our forefathers used to eat and what they used to take in the form of medicines, we can reconstruct certain vital ingredients in the healthy artery equation.

But before looking at this far healthier picture, it may be useful to see how far we as individuals have strayed from it. So first, the bad news. What follows is a list of contributory factors to arterial disease. Tick your score.

ARTERIAL DISEASE FACTORS

● Overweight

● Bouts of energetic exercise rather than consistent exercise

● Stress, especially bottled anger

● Smoking (increases risk of arterial disease by 70 per cent)

● Alcohol (more than two drinks a day)

● High blood lipids (usually caused by too many fats in diet)

● High uric acid levels (caused by high protein diets – the 'good' life)

● Too much salt – 3gm (0.03oz) a day is all that is needed (the average person eats 10 times more than this)

● Too much sugar (the average person consumes more than 50kg (112lb) a year – think of that in terms of bags of sugar)

● Too little fibre (fibre binds with fat and helps clear it)

● Low intake of vitamins, especially vitamins A, C and E (these act as free-radical scavengers, putting them out of action)

● Low intake of minerals, especially magnesium, chromium and selenium, three vital minerals for arterial health one of which, magnesium, is not present in sufficient quantities in the average British diet. The food consumed in many countries of the world is now often grown on soils deficient in selenium and other vital trace minerals.

● Family history of arterial disease

This list has been adapted from a wonderful booklet by British nutritional expert Patrick Holford called *Super Nutrition for a Healthy Heart* (see Useful Addresses. If you live elsewhere, write to your local Heart Foundation for information, or choose one of the many titles in your local health bookstore, under the general heading Arterial Disease and Diet.)

REDRESSING THE DAMAGE: THE GOOD NEWS

There are many ways in which arterial damage can be reversed, and they can be taken by every individual. Here are some of them.

DIETARY DIRECTIONS
Follow the 12 golden rules of healthy digestion found in Chapter 4, omitting no. 12 if circulatory problems exist. Also read about food combining and cooking food the energetic way.

To this dietary advice, add the following, which are specifically for those believing they may have a circulatory disorder or have a family history of it.

● Eliminate shellfish and fish roe, which are too high in cholesterol.

● Avoid fatty nuts such as cashews, Brazils and macadamias. Eat instead a few almonds or seeds such as sesame or sunflower.

● Reduce your intake of dairy products to 100g (4oz) of butter a week (cut it off and keep it separate), 225g (8oz) of cheese a week (chosen from Edam, Gouda fromage frais, quark, or skimmed milk cottage) and 300ml ($\frac{1}{2}$ pt) of skimmed milk a day (including all uses such as in tea and coffee).

● Eat wholemeal or rye bread (maximum three slices a day) or a few crispbread slices, oat or water biscuits.

● Use fresh wholemeal pasta (no greasy, meaty sauces) but even better is buckwheat pasta or brown rice.

● Eat avocados, butter squash, potatoes (especially sweet) and other high-calorie foods sparingly, especially if you are overweight.

● Eat more fish than meat (approximately 100g/4 oz a day of either). If meat, favour lean lamb, veal or free-range poultry, dry-roasted or steamed (with the skin cut off). The best fish is that rich in the HDL oils your system needs in order to control cholesterol levels – halibut, fresh salmon, herrings, mackerel, fresh sardines or a few anchovies, for example.

● Eggs are high in cholesterol, so best limit these to two or three small free-range eggs a week.

● To the breakfasts suggested in Chapter 4 add 20ml (2 tablespoons) of lecithin granules. This helps to keep cholesterol in suspension and away from arterial deposits, just as detergents keep fats in suspension.

● Eat at least 10ml (1 tablespoon) oats and oatbran daily.
(Read more about why in Robert Kowalski's book, referenced in Chapter 1.)

NUTRITIONAL NUTS AND BOLTS
To the nutritional advice given in Chapter 4, add the following:

● One concentrated E.P.A. tablet daily of 180mg

● In addition, gamma linolenic acid (commonly in the form of oil of evening primrose); 500mg can be taken

● Some circulatory disorders favourably respond to supplementation of the B group of vitamins, particularly B_3 (niacin or nicotinic acid) and B_6 (pyrodoxine), a mild diuretic. Until or unless nutritional advice is sought, these are best taken daily in the form of a general B supplement, since all vitamins work synergistically (together).

Make sure the vitamin/mineral supplement you choose (see Chapter 4) contains adequate magnesium (at least 200mg). There is a strong association between magnesium deficiency and heart disease risks. This mineral helps to prevent muscular spasms, which can be serious if arteries are narrowed. Other minerals that should be represented in your supplement include selenium, zinc, manganese, potassium and calcium. Co-Q-10 is a vital nutrient for heart health, since it improves the cells' ability to use oxygen, which is also helpful if arteries are narrowed and blood supply restricted.

In a combined trial carried out by University of Austin, Texas, and the Centre for Adult Diseases in Osaka, Japan, 52 patients with high blood pressure were treated either with Co-Q or with placebo tablets. There was a decrease of 11 per cent in blood pressure for those on Co-Q and of only 2 per cent for those on the placebo. In the past few years no fewer than 20 trials have repeatedly demonstrated its remarkable ability, and 12 million people in Japan now take it.

In a book of this kind there is not room to go into nutritional dosage details, which will vary from person to person anyway, nor would it be appropriate to suggest individual supplements. However there is much information about dosages in the previously mentioned booklet, by Patrick Holford.

There is another booklet published by the UK Arterial Disease Foundation, written by Richard Brown, himself a survivor of several heart attacks and an advocate of alternative ways of dealing with this problem, especially chelation (see below). Details of this are also given in Useful Addresses. These two booklets make a wonderful duo of 'complementary' advice about arterial health. Both can be read in an hour.

SMOKING, STIMULANTS AND CIRCULATORY DISORDERS
All stimulants – nicotine, coffee, tea, pep pills, soft drinks containing caffeine and so on – work by increasing blood pressure, and many cause arterial constriction as well. This is not good news for anyone whose arteries are already narrowed by arterial disease.

Smoking a packet of cigarettes a day gives you twice the risk of heart attack and five times the risk of a stroke. Please read the section in Chapter 6 about giving up, even if you have tried to give up before. At least the information there will help you to understand the addiction, and once something is understood it is easier to tackle.

EASING THE HEART-FELT BURDEN OF STRESS AND HYPERVENTILATION
Stress is bad news for any body system: the vital circulatory system

suffers more than most. Useful ways of controlling stress are suggested in Chapter 7. In Chapter 6 (Respiration) the stress-reaction of hyperventilation is discussed (because it is a breathing disorder), but it is one that concerns itself equally with the circulatory system because of the intimate connection between the lungs and breathing, and heart rate. When one increases so does the other, and vice versa.

Doctors believe that hyperventilation – chest-centred over-breathing as a response to fear, anger or other stressors – is the cause of many unpleasant symptoms experienced by their 'heart' patients, including impaired concentration or dizziness through to memory lapses, speech anomalies, disturbances of vision or even complete unconsciousness. Simple techniques for learning to re-breathe more naturally are suggested, together with explanations about why this habit can be so draining. If you have a tendency to gasp when under stress or take in air quickly through your mouth, you probably hyperventilate from time to time.

CHELATION: A HEART-LIFTING THERAPY

For those who know already that they have a circulatory system condition, is there any other solution besides permanently taking drugs such as beta-blockers, living low-key lifestyles or having by-pass surgery? There is indeed – and it is the up-and-coming treatment of the future, available now through a medically-supervised world-wide network whose addresses are published in Richard Brown's booklet.

This treatment, chelation, is a highly successful and safe way of eliminating arterial plaque, otherwise known as atheroma, a word appropriately derived from the Greek word for porridge.

Chelation happens to be derived from another Greek word, 'chele', meaning the grasping claw of a crab or lobster, and this derivation gives a clue to what the process actually does: in effect, it 'grabs' or 'claws' the arterial plaque from the arterial walls in much the same way as a dry cleaning solvent extracts stains from fabric surfaces.

In fact, the substance used to chelate plaque from arteries, a kind of man-made amino acid called EDTA (ethylene diamine tetra-acetic acid) was first used for that very purpose – to remove calcium stains from fabrics. Then some lateral thinking made some scientists realize its value as a chelator, not only of calcium but of poisonous metals such as lead from the body. Chelators increase the solubility of a substance thus making it more bio-available, in this case, for elimination through the bloodstream and urinary functions.

People with lead poisoning treated in this way were seen to improve dramatically as well because calcium deposits were removed from arterial plaque, and it was from these observations that EDTA's application to arterial disease was developed.

Since its introduction in the early 1950s over 4 million chelation treatments have been given in the USA, 20,000 in Australia, plus several thousand in Holland and more recently in the UK. In all that time, despite recipients being very often desperately ill and given up by their doctors, *there has never been a death directly related to the therapy.*

The empirical evidence of its benefits is overwhelming. There are hundreds of written testimonials from patients of all ages who have experienced sometimes dramatic improvements in their symptoms after chelation therapy. For many people having been refused by-pass surgery because their arteries were too fragile or their health too poor this treatment has been the last hope.

Improvements noted include less fatigue on exertion, more mental alertness, less angina (heart pain), reduction in blood pressure and improvement in conditions such as osteoporosis (surprisingly the process does not 'claw' calcium from the bones but actually promotes better calcium metabolism).

Chelation is done on an outpatient basis. EDTA is given as an intravenous drip or infusion, each treatment lasting between 3 and 4 hours, during which time the patient listens to music, chats to other patients, eats, drinks or whatever.

Most patients take themselves home afterwards. Between ten and twenty treatments are the average requirement, but there is often marked improvement after five.

The substance is eliminated from the body within 24 hours, so there is no accumulation. However, the kidneys, organs of elimination (see Chapter 10), must be checked before a course of treatment is started. In the past, when this precaution was not taken, kidney damage sometimes occurred. This does not happen now, partly because of the precautionary tests, and partly because a lower and better regulated dose of EDTA is given.

The benefits of chelation are obvious – in clearing the entire arterial system of its plaque, blood supply to every organ is improved, so the body's job of nourishing its tissues and removing waste products is facilitated. When there are more than 48,000km (30,000 miles) of arterial tubing in the body and an amazing 10,000,000,000 capillaries, it is hardly feasible to suppose that plaque forms only on those arteries feeding the heart, the brain and the legs, the prime sites where symptoms are suffered. It is simply that in those areas the effects are more serious and surgical intervention is often life-saving, such as in bypass surgery, which clears one or two centimetres (just under 1in) of arteries of the heart.

In this context bypass surgery can be seen as the emergency measure it undoubtedly is. Clinical trials are now being done to fulfil medical establishment requirements, but it seems they will find out little that is not already empirically known and observed – after all, the substance EDTA has been tried and tested since the 1930s – unlike some drugs such as Opren and Halcion, which passed clinical trials, only to be withdrawn once sufficient empirical evidence was gathered as to their dangers.

An additional benefit of intravenous chelation is thought to accrue from the fact that the process sweeps up molecules of lead, aluminium (a key factor in Alzheimer's disease), copper, iron and other metals deposited abnormally throughout the body by middle age and before. Mercury is another deadly poison, and 'silver' dental amalgam contains no less than 40 per cent of this deadly ingredient, some of which 'leaks' into the system (see Chapter 8, Teeth). Raised copper levels are often seen in those who take the contraceptive pill. Zinc supplements, given with chelation therapy, also aid in the removal of these metals, especially aluminium.

THE NATURAL CHELATORS

Nature has provided us with natural chelators in the form of vitamins and minerals, in particular vitamins A, C and E and the minerals magnesium, selenium and zinc – which is why it is so important to have a healthy diet supplemented by a wise nutritional programme.

ROAD CHECKING YOUR CIRCULATORY SYSTEM

Since World War II many people have lived on a diet of processed food. In the 1940s and 1950s it was thought that we needed lots of protein for health. Protein was regarded as a wonder food, and early weight-reducing diets usually concentrated on high-protein, low-starch regimes. These two misconceptions are almost invariably key factors in today's epidemic of arterial-related diseases.

We are now learning by our mistakes, but the damage has, at least for several generations, been done, and our inheritance from earlier errors must now be dealt with by having regular check-ups.

Both blood pressure and blood lipid (fat) levels should be checked annually, especially if there is a family history of CHD. Holford's booklet contains guides to what safe results should be. Doctors may or may not offer you this information to which you are, after all, entitled. Considering the numbers of patients doctors have to care for, it makes sense to keep an eye on these details for yourself, not to do their job for them but to see that their job is made easier by your checking in on time. There are also home cholesterol testing kits to aid you in your endeavours.

THERAPIES FOR A HEALTHY HEART

Apart from those measures mentioned in connection with lowering stress levels, the technique of reflexology is particularly suited to those with coronary disorders, since massaging the feet helps to clear the circulatory system and to stimulate the elimination of unwanted substances from the blood. It is also very relaxing – those with circulatory disorders are often high-achievers and need this kind of measure. Read about it in Chapter 8.

Above all, never feel that it is too late to redress circulatory disorders: this system responds very quickly to effort.

6
*

THE RESPIRATORY SYSTEM

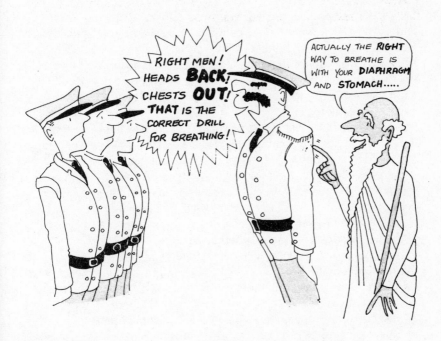

IN THIS CHAPTER

✱ New kind of breath test ✱ System workings – easy as
breathing ✱ Why we need trees ✱ Cough protection
mechanism ✱ Exploring lung capacity ✱ Conquering colds
and flu ✱ Understanding asthma ✱ Staying on top of hay
fever ✱ Positively the last word on giving up smoking ✱ Dire
consequences of overbreathing ✱ Learning to breathe: how to
save yourself 4,000 breaths a day

EXERCISE: TAKING A BREATH TEST

Before starting to read this chapter, consider for a moment your own breathing. Are you breathing through your nose or your mouth? Is your chest doing most of the moving or is your abdomen doing it? Are your breaths even, or do you gasp from time to time or sigh a lot? Is your inhalation longer than your exhalation or vice versa? You may have to catch yourself at it several times before you get all your breathing patterns identified, but note them down; they will be of value later.

Now think back. As a child, were you told to 'stick your chest out and keep your tummy flat'? Nearly all of us were. You think this is natural? At the earliest opportunity, watch a baby breathe. This will leave you in no doubt that a baby breathes naturally from its stomach while most adults breathe with their chests. This appalling indoctrinated habit causes us to take, on average, 4,000 more breaths a day than a stomach-breather.

Quite apart from that, chest breathing signifies to the body that we are aroused, we are preparing for a challenge. It is a good way of getting air into the lungs quickly when, for example, we need it for exercise or when we wake up in the morning, but otherwise it keeps us in a permanent state of red alert. Doctors say it leads to one of the most health-debilitating habits of all time – hyperventilation or overbreathing (see below). Suffice to say, it is a habit people get into which keeps them permanently stressed, at least when awake.

How has this happened, when breathing – respiration – is one of the most automatic things we do? Phrases in our language reflect this simplicity – 'as easy as breathing', 'as normal as drawing a breath' and so on.

It is only when things go wrong and it becomes hard to breathe because of a shortage of air or a chest infection that we realize how vital to life, second by second, breathing is.

Try holding your breath and you will see the truth of it. Automatic body reflexes simply take over after a very short space of time and force you to breathe. A body process as vital as breathing simply cannot lapse: 3 minutes without oxygen and brain cells die, the heart struggles to keep beating, its muscle starved from lack of oxygen, so that within a few more minutes the body reaches a point of no return – or a point at which, if there is a return, vital systems will have been irreparably damaged.

Healthwise, one of our biggest disadvantages is that breathing comes naturally. Not only do we take its process for granted, but we assume the process is working efficiently, when all it may be doing is working sufficiently to keep us alive. And that is not all: not only does the respiratory system suffer from our poor breathing techniques, but it also suffers from lack of maintenance.

We change the filters on our air conditioners and on the air intake systems on our cars quite regularly, but we never stop to consider whether we are cleansing and conditioning our own respiratory system. In fact, smokers actually defy the system to function in spite of their efforts to clog it!

THE WHYS AND WHEREFORES OF RESPIRATION

The respiratory system, which consists of nose, windpipe, bronchial tubes and lungs, is there for one major reason – all body cells need oxygen in order to convert ('burn') food into energy for life. In doing so they give off carbon dioxide as a waste product, so the function of respiration is to allow the uptake of oxygen from the air into the blood and to permit carbon dioxide to be lost from the blood back into the air.

On paper this seems simple, but anyone who tries to dissolve oxygen in water will quickly see that it is not readily soluble: bubbles of it simply stream through the liquid and disappear out again. Since blood is largely water, it seems unfeasible for this to happen.

In fact, the body achieves it by an ingenious reversible process. The red corpuscles in the blood are red because of haemoglobin. This remarkable pigment is a combination of haem (an iron-porphyrin compound) and globin (a protein). Haemoglobin binds with oxygen at the comparatively high pressures found inside the lung tissues and is then able to release oxygen again at the lower pressure found in the body tissues. The high levels of carbon dioxide and acid present in these active tissues as a result of their energy-producing activity further promote the release of oxygen.

Then, by another chemical process, the carbon dioxide combines with the water in the red corpuscles (carbon dioxide is 20 times more soluble than oxygen) and is transported back to the lungs, where, under the different pressure existing there, it is released.

The whole principle of the exchange of gases in the lungs is made possible by diffusion in response to differences in pressure. A gas always diffuses from an area where its pressure is high to an area where its pressure is low. That the whole process takes place in milliseconds is another body miracle.

Obviously the ease with which oxygen is taken up by the haemoglobin depends on the quality of the blood: this is why iron is such an important factor in diet, since it is a vital constituent of haemoglobin. Various degrees of anaemia can exist unrecognized in the body, especially in menstruating women, affecting this vital process. So foods rich in iron, such as red meats, eggs, parsley, spinach and watercress etc. plus, if necessary, 25mg iron daily, should be taken. (Vegetarians need to be especially vigilant in iron intake as vegetable sources of iron are not as bio-available as animal sources.) Never take iron with tea; it will block its absorption.

WHY 'SAVE OURSELVES' MEANS 'SAVE OUR TREES'

With every living creature breathing out carbon dioxide and taking up oxygen, the Earth's supply of oxygen would soon be depleted were it not for the compensatory fact that trees and vegetation do the reverse – they take up carbon dioxide and give off oxygen. This is why it is so vital to preserve our rain forests (additionally because they keep the water balance stable). The simple fact is that without trees we die, and the situation is becoming critical. This is why we all feel better in the country, where the air balance supports us better. City dwellers profit by having living plants in the house, or better still, if they have a garden, planting as many trees as they can.

THE WORKINGS OF THE RESPIRATORY SYSTEM

Air enters the body through the nose, which contains special shelf-like projections which act like radiator baffles to warm and moisten the air so that it is not such a shock to the system. Breathing through the mouth is a very bad habit and should happen only when extra air is needed for exercise and exertion.

Passing through the larynx – a complex valve, which rides up when swallowing food (check by swallowing now) to prevent its entry into the air passages – the air then passes into the trachea or windpipe. This looks just like some commercial hoses and is reinforced by rings of cartilage, which can be felt in the neck. The trachea also acts as an air filter in that it is lined with fine hairs which produce mucus to trap any dust particles, which by these means are swept up to the larynx, to be coughed out.

THE COUGH REFLEX

The cough is one of the most important protective reflexes contained in the body, without which many things could lodge in the windpipe and cause suffocation. Coughing also enables us to eject bacteria, irritants and excess mucus. The cough reflex is so powerful that air evacuated in this way can actually reach the speed of sound!

The trachea divides under the breastbone, sending branches to both lungs. This is the first of no fewer than 16 branchings by which the bronchi, as they are now called, divide and sub-divide into smaller and smaller 'twigs' – estimates suggest there may be up to an amazing 650,000 of them.

On the end of these twigs are the operative parts of the lungs, where the respiratory bronchioles open into grape-like clusters of thin-walled sacs, called alveoli. The total surface area of the alveoli has been estimated as falling between 50 and 75sq m (60–90sq yd), although at birth it is only a fraction of this – 3–4sq m (3.5–5sq yd). Put another way, there are between 300,000,000 and 400,000,000 alveoli in the lungs.

These alveoli are covered in a network of fine capillaries containing blood. Air and blood are in contact across the thin walls, only two cells thick, and here, and only here, does exchange of gases by diffusion occur. The rest of the lung is simply for getting the right ingredients together. However it is no less vital: if airways get blocked, the vital gases cannot be exchanged.

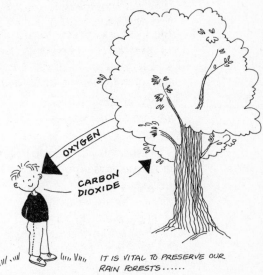

IT IS VITAL TO PRESERVE OUR RAIN FORESTS......

AIR CIRCULATION THROUGH THE BLOOD

The oxygenated blood from these capillary networks feeds into larger and larger veins running through the lung tissue until eventually it leaves the lungs in the pulmonary veins (see Chapter 5, Circulation) and is returned to the atrium on the left side of the heart to be pumped through the aorta to the entire body system, thus giving the cells their vital supply of oxygen. From the tissues, the blood then picks up carbon dioxide and other cell waste materials, returning it through the veins into the right side of the heart to be pumped back to the lungs for the cycle to begin again.

THE MECHANICS OF BREATHING

The functioning of the lungs resembles that of a pair of bellows. The muscles of the diaphragm and chest wall pull the lung 'bellows' apart, and air is drawn in; then they relax and air passes out. To achieve this activity, the lungs have to be isolated in an air-tight cavity, called the thorax, of which the ribs, intercostal muscles, sternum, diaphragm and upper section of the spine are all parts.

The mechanics of breathing, even to this day, are not fully understood. The movements of breathing continue independently of will, and yet they are also subject to it, as well as to changes in the body and in the surrounding environment. What is known is that cells in the brainstem at the base of the brain are closely involved in establishing the rhythm and depth of breathing. These cells appear to be sensitive not so much to the oxygen levels in the blood as to carbon dioxide levels. However they are also affected by impulses from the higher, 'thinking' part of the brain so that thoughts and emotions can affect breathing too. It is a system that works on feedback, and the feedback comes from both physical sources, such as the stimulus of exercise or pain, and psychological sources, such as fear, joy or indignation. All these emotions affect breathing, as anyone who has ever taken (or held) a breath in the grips of one or other of them knows.

LUNG CAPACITY

The capacity of the lung to respond to demands for oxygen by the tissues, during exercise, for example, can increase to more than 20 times its resting rate – that is, instead of ingesting the average 7 litres ($1\frac{1}{2}$ gallons) of air per minute it can ingest up to 150 litres (33 gallons) per minute! The sight of an athlete coming off the track, unable to talk for a few minutes until the enormous rate of breathing slows down from the exercising to the resting body's needs, is a graphic illustration of this response. Such exercise, of course, strengthens the lungs enormously, enabling them to cope better with the task of eliminating one of the plagues of 20th-century life – air pollution. In fact, in a test, an athlete walking around New York city area returned with very little evidence of having inhaled polluted air – his lung function had been strong enough to expel it.

THE CHALLENGE OF THE 20TH CENTURY TO HEALTHY LUNGS

The past 20 years have not unfolded a pretty picture as far as lung disease is concerned. Doctors agree that in that period there has been an alarming increase in the incidence of lung cancer, chronic bronchitis and emphysema, as well as in industrial lung disease. If this trend increases we could all be faced with a very serious situation, and there is every indication that it will continue, because the factors affecting it are also increasing. Personal awareness coupled with effort is the only solution. Here is a profile of what is happening.

Air pollution is on the increase, partly because industrialization is on the increase and partly because not enough sanctions are being taken against those who are pumping the trillions of gallons of sulphur dioxide and other pollutants such as chlorofluorocarbons (CFCs) from aerosols and hydrocarbons from car exhausts into the air. There is a saturation point and we are nearing it. As usual, big business is resisting taking steps that will trim their profits but individuals are also resisting, by continuing to use aerosols and to drive cars that do not have catalytic converters or that have not been converted to use lead-free petrol.

WHERE THERE'S SMOKE, THERE'S FIRE

However doctors agree that at present cigarette smoke is still *the* major contributor to the increase in lung diseases, and that this affects passive smokers – those who just inhale other people's smoke – as well as active smokers, of whom an alarming proportion are young, child-bearing women. For new insight into giving up, see the section on tackling smoking.

Lung disease may be caused by physical factors such as dust and pollutants in the air, by bacteria and viruses, by sensitivity phenomena, such as occur in asthma, or by disorders in the circulating blood – lungs are a prime site, for example, for secondaries from malignant disease elsewhere in the body. The importance of taking seriously any early sign of lung dysfunction cannot be overemphasized, yet incredibly we take medication to suppress these early warning signs, such as coughing. We also try to suppress the symptoms of colds, which mask from us the extent to which the condition of our lungs may have deteriorated from their normal, healthy strength. Obviously, a balance has to be struck between coughing oneself half to death with a cold or flu and taking medication, but it is important to be aware of what the body is trying to draw attention to – that the lung capacity is probably depleted and there is need for rest. The eloquence of body symptoms lies in their perfect demonstration of the principle, 'a stitch in time saves nine'.

Thus frequent colds may indicate that general resistance is low, or lowering, or that lung health may not be sufficient to expel more serious foreign invaders.

COUGH ALERT

Any persistent cough should never be overlooked. Anyone with a cough, however slight, especially in the early mornings, could have the early symptoms of bronchitis. Anyone with a history of asthma from childhood should not just rely on inhalers to clear the air passages (as these work less and less efficiently as time goes by), but should look at their diet and lifestyle (see section on asthma).

COLDS AND FLU PROTECTION PLAN

This plan is also a good insurance policy against ME, which often starts with a viral infection.

Many studies have shown that catching cold bears very little relation to being exposed to cold germs, which are present in the air at any time. However, it does bear relation to being under par, at which time being in close proximity to anyone with a cold will have inevitable results. There is also a sympathy element involved, whether from being got down by the other person's misery or by concern is hard to divine! We are complex creatures.

Building up immunity to colds can save you from an insidious chain reaction whereby catching colds frequently further lowers resistance until ultimately a much more serious infection such as one of the strains of flu is caught, with the danger of post-viral infection or ME as an aftermath.

It simply isn't worth taking this risk when studies have shown that it is so easy to build up immunity to colds by the simple procedure of regularly – that is, daily – taking vitamin C. Vitamin C alone is not enough, however. For ideal protection bioflavinoids should be taken as well, since they work with vitamin C to protect the body from infection. Extra supplies of zinc are needed too, especially if a cold is just beginning. However, no one mineral or vitamin should ever be taken on its own, since they all work synergistically – in conjunction with each other. Hence a multi-vitamin and mineral tablet should be taken daily in conjunction with vitamin C and citrus bioflavinoids.

COLDS, STRESS AND VITAMIN C THERAPY

Of the people in one small London study who were selected because they suffered from frequent colds, 81 per cent of those who followed the regime of taking vitamin C reported improved immunity, and 52 per cent reported faster recovery if they did contract a cold. An interesting factor revealed in the study was the fact that people were more likely to catch colds if they had just undergone a major event in their lives such as marriage, divorce, new job or bereavement. The new science of psychoneurimmunology (see Chapters 7 and 11) has demonstrated only too clearly the web of interconnectedness between body, mind and the emotions, but that needs be of no great consequence so long as we intervene at one of the physical points to prevent such effects on health from completely undermining us so that we contract the really serious complication of a 20th-century disease.

Individual requirements for vitamin C vary enormously, but one thing is certain: recommended or required daily allowances (RDAs) should be completely ignored. These merely set a level below which signs of vitamin C deficiency, such as scurvy, would show themselves. To live on RDAs is a bit like living on a diet sufficient to keep us alive, just above starvation level.

There is one clear way of testing how much vitamin C each individual needs and that is to take increasing amounts of it until the bowels become loose. Just under this amount is the right quantity of vitamin C needed daily. This level may be so amazingly high as to be prohibitive in terms of both cost and consumption (Linus Pauling, a key discoverer of the connection between infections and vitamin C levels, used to take 17gm a day). A safe minimum would be to take 1gm a day, increasing to 3 or more grams at the earliest sign of a cold. People in the study reported that they had immunity to colds for up to 3 months after taking their tablets. However, it should also be said that it took about that long to build up the required immunity level, so starting well before the winter is wise. Vitamin C also protects us against a variety of 20th-century ills, such as pollution, stress, infection, and damage caused by drinking. Smokers can also benefit by increasing their vitamin C, since the actual smoking habit uses up many times more vitamin C than non-smokers require.

INFLUENZA AND THE RESPIRATORY SYSTEM

Compared to colds, strains of flu, of which there are three or four, are far more serious, because they attack not only the respiratory system but other systems as well. Tremendous multiplication of the flu virus occurs within the initial 24-hour period, which is why early signs should be acknowledged and not defied, as so many people try to do by staying on their feet.

The severe epidemic of 1918–19 was one of the worst catastrophes on record, and it is estimated that more than 20 million people died around the world. In 1957 there was another terrible epidemic, in which the Asian (type A) strain was involved. Epidemics tends to go in 3-year cycles, some worse than others, and having had flu does not guarantee lasting immunity, as the virus can mutate, and immunity is specific to type. Nonetheless, if an epidemic seems to be on the way, once the strain of flu causing it has been identified, it certainly pays to be immunized. But the best immunization is to build up the body's immune system by eating the right foods and supplementing with the body's chief protective vitamins such as C, E and A.

LUNGS AND ALLERGIES

Unfortunately the lungs are particularly liable to involvement in allergic responses, which feature today in the enormously increasing incidence of asthma and hay fever, especially among city dwellers. These conditions, if not addressed, can lead to impaired lung function or at the very best shallow breathing habits, undermining body energy which depends on oxygen and impairing healthy defences.

CHECK YOUR CHEST

Regular – annual – lung-performance checks and chest X-rays at recommended intervals should be part and parcel of any health-screening programme. Lung function is important, because vital energy levels depend upon it. Lung power improves tremendously (and quickly) with just 10 minutes' aerobic exercise a day – swimming, jogging, re-bounding, skipping, dancing – or just running up the stairs instead of using the elevator.

IMPROVING YOUR DOMESTIC AIR SUPPLY

City dwellers can benefit enormously from buying an air purifier, which is quite different from an air conditioner. This comparatively inexpensive piece of equipment, sold in most large department stores or advertised in health catalogues, will not only clean and filter the air inside your home, removing microscopic dust particles, pollen and smoke, but will also balance the energy-draining positive 'charge' in city air.

This is achieved by the incorporation of an ionizer, which produces invigorating negative ions. This creates an environment similar to that occurring in places we find refreshing such as on mountains and near to waterfalls and the sea, all of which areas have high levels of negative ions.

Closer to cities these levels become drastically reduced, because of smoke, traffic pollution, air conditioning units and the static charges that develop from synthetic materials, including carpets, and from television and computer screens.

Regular cleaning of the ionizer 'head' within the air purifier is necessary, as is changing its filters, and one sight of these after a few months' use will convince anyone of their protective capacity.

ASTHMA AND HAY FEVER

As the 20th century progressed and psychology became more and more fashionable (there are fashions in health and medicine just as there are elsewhere) allergic responses such as asthma were increasingly attributed to emotional sources. Now it is realized that the picture is far more complex, and diet is being increasingly investigated as a cause as are environmental factors.

Any mucus-forming foods, such as dairy products, should be eliminated from the diet of an asthmatic. Two other prime likely allergens are wheat and eggs. Allergens are nearly always staple foods in the diet which are commonly, if not daily eaten.

Allergies affecting the respiratory system, such as asthma and hay fever, are made all the more serious because they are prejudicing one of the body's vital processes, breathing. They are also the more serious in that they often involve children who are at the key growing stage of their lives, when anything that depletes or erodes body energy could have long-lasting ramifications. In fact one survey of students attending 514 schools in the UK revealed that just under 15 per cent of children suffered badly from the effects of hay fever. This was reflected in lowered performance of no less than 43 per cent of them when taking key exams. Regrettably hay fever reaches its peak in June, which is exam time in the northern hemisphere.

Often misdiagnosed as a summer cold (and therefore left untreated), hay fever is an allergic reaction largely affecting the nose and eyes, although it is sometimes associated with asthma and other allergic conditions. Pollens, particularly of ragweed, mugwort and oilseed rape, are chiefly to blame, especially in the case of seasonal hay fever, but tree pollens and mould spores also play a key role. It is also suspected that modern pollutants play their part, as hay fever as we know it now was yet another affliction virtually unheard of before the turn of this century.

To understand what is going on, one needs to understand a bit more about the mechanics of allergy. Allergy actually involves part of the body's defences or immune responses. Not only does the body fight bacteria and viruses, but it also protects itself from protein substances such as pollens and moulds, recognizing them as foreign. It reacts against air-borne chemicals as well.

Marshalling its defences involves the very T-cells that have become so well known to the public since the onset of another immune-related disease, AIDS. Over-stressing the T-cells by putting them constantly in a state of attack, withdraw, attack can lead to their exhaustion, when they will either over-react or not react at all.

TESTING YOUR ZINC LEVELS

The balance between the two types of T-cells, which turn on and off the immune system reaction, is controlled partly by nutrition and partly by hormonal activity, which indirectly depends on good nutrition, too. Zinc is one mineral that is vital to the functioning of the immune response, and it is known that the average British diet simply does not contain enough of this vital mineral. The same is probably true of the United States, since they, too, eat enormous quantities of fast food.

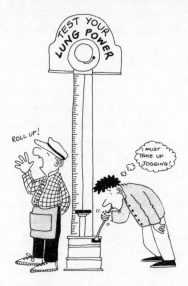

There is a product available in the UK market called Zincatest. This tells you to take a certain dosage – if you can taste it, you are not zinc deficient; if you cannot taste it, you most certainly are. Zinc affects both taste and smell, so those who feel these senses are diminishing should suspect depleted zinc levels and test themselves.

WHAT TO DO FOR HAY FEVER

Hay fever is really an early warning sign from your body that your immune system is under stress, otherwise your mucous membranes would have been strong enough to stop the pollen from getting into the bloodstream.

However, since they are there, careful selection of drops, measures and medication to control the symptoms seems reasonable. Teachers say that many children suffer untreated hay fever symptoms, which definitely affect their concentration between spring and autumn.

SHORT-TERM STRATEGIES

Close all windows, especially in the morning, and in the car. Repeat this procedure in the evenings, especially at dusk. Keep sufferers' bedrooms free of dust, and keep pets away from them – some effects compound each other. Cut down on all processed foods, sugary foods, chocolate, fizzy drinks, oranges, milk and milk products (except live yoghurt), highly-coloured foods (unless completely natural) and potato crisps. Drink only bottled water.

Medications include:

1. Antihistamines. These reduce the body's defence reaction and should be taken only in the short term. It should also be borne in mind that they almost invariably make one drowsy.
2. Steroids. These are given for severe cases of asthma and hay fever. Their side-effects and long-term effects on the body are so serious, especially affecting the normal growth of children, that they should be viewed only as an emergency measure. If they are prescribed, do try and see a doctor who specializes in natural ways of combating allergies.
3. Sodium cromolglycate. This was discovered in the 1960s and is thought to be one of the safest drugs that can be given for asthma and hay fever. It is important that it is taken regularly to prevent symptoms recurring. It is most helpful when included in eye drops to relieve eye irritation. A combination of the nasal spray beclomethsone and eyedrops of sodium cromolglycate came out top of one study involving 140 general practitioners for controlling hay fever symptoms.
4. Desensitization. This is a form of treatment which is helpful only when the actual cause – pollen or spore – is known. Injections are prepared which stimulate antibody production in the body. The effect is good in the short term, but often the allergy changes to another allergen and the whole process has to be repeated; in other words, none of these things is curing the complaint, they are just controlling the symptoms.
5. Vasoconstrictor sprays (such as ephedrine and xylometrazoline). These should be used with great reluctance since there is a rebound effect which becomes a vicious circle, with less and less relief and more and more need.

LONG-TERM STRATEGIES
These involve the acknowledgement that the body's defences must be built up. Diet must be examined, with real attention paid to fresh, unchemicalized, additive-free food.

It is sometimes necessary to go on a desensitizing diet, such as the lamb and pears diet. Any professional allergy dietary adviser will explain the steps and why.

Other stressors need to be examined and tested to see if they are contributing to the overload. This can be done quite simply and harmlessly by a practitioner skilled in using kineseology (muscle testing – see Useful Addresses and read about it in Chapter 12). In this way foods can be tested, as can any medications or household items and chemicals used by the sufferer, including the local tap water. Soon, there will be a profile of the worst offenders, substitutions for which can generally be found.

Constipation is another cause of toxins building up in the body, which have then to be excreted by secondary means, such as through the skin or through the mucous membranes. The weakening effect that this has on these secondary lines of defence in the body leads to complaints of these tissues. Chapter 4 will be helpful in suggesting natural steps to cure constipation.

Finally there is the question of locality. If the allergic person lives near a main road or a chemical factory or in some other area where commercial pollutants or other factors may be contaminating the local atmosphere (including nuclear plants and high tension wires), serious consideration may have to be given to moving to another area. The benefits from such vigilance will not only apply to a recession of the allergy symptoms, but to health improvements in general.

TACKLING THE SMOKING HABIT

Nearly everyone who smokes wants to give up. Most will have tried, once or many times with varying success. Some will have tried a technique, such as hypnotherapy or acupuncture, to help them in their endeavours.

Most smokers are aware of the horrifying statistics, and having them thrust at them does not help one little bit. So this section is not going to thrust statistics at readers; the most it will do in this vein is to give some information about what is inhaled in smoke that many smokers do not know about. If you do not want to read that bit, skip it, but do read about the reasons about why it is so hard to give up, why hypnotherapy and aversion therapy and even acupuncture, while succeeding in many instances in enabling you to give up for a time, do not enable you to give up permanently. That requires understanding what is behind the subconscious desire to smoke, acknowledging that package of information and knowingly taking it on board.

IS IT ADDICTION?

Certainly smoking is an addiction, but the addiction is not so much to nicotine as to a habit, a habit that is probably attached to a series of mind sets. Tests have proved beyond doubt that nicotine actually leaves the body within 24 hours of stopping smoking, and there is often no real awareness from smokers of whether they have nicotine in their systems or not. This has been shown by other tests that have secretly introduced nicotine into the bloodstreams of smokers wanting to give up to see if it made their withdrawal easier – it didn't. So it was not the nicotine they were missing. This is not to deny that nicotine is a powerful drug, but it seems that it was the *habit* of smoking that was most difficult to break.

WHAT HAPPENS WHEN A SMOKER LIGHTS UP

Many smokers say that the first cigarette in the morning is the best; some say a cigarette after a period when they could not smoke is the best. The fact is that nicotine gives the smoker a buzz when it is first inhaled. The longer it is since the last buzz, the stronger the sensation – hence the first cigarette of the day feeling. The physical responses attending this buzz are that the heart beats faster for a few minutes, adrenalin is released into the bloodstream and the blood vessels constrict. This adds to the buzz – the feeling that the body is getting ready to do something, which it is.

What has been activated is the fight or flight reflex (see Chapter 7). This is a tensing, energy-using reflex, which cannot be continued forever without the body getting drained – relaxation must alternate with it. Thus smoking, while appearing to release energy, actually drains it.

WHERE THERE'S SMOKE, THERE'S ONLY FIRE!

Smoke is not food, nor is it oxygen, both of which replenish energy to the body, because they are the building blocks of energy. Smoking a cigarette is simply drawing on the body's energy bank by making it work harder. After each cigarette will come a compensatory dip in energy while the body recovers its equilibrium, and that is when the smoker lights up again – to bring the energy back to the level at which it was.

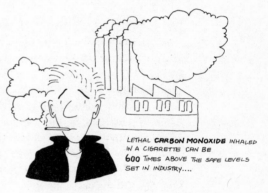

LETHAL **CARBON MONOXIDE** INHALED IN A CIGARETTE CAN BE **600** TIMES ABOVE THE SAFE LEVELS SET IN INDUSTRY....

Another buzz, but no energy created, only energy lost. Although the heart beats faster, which should deliver more oxygen for energy to the tissues, there is, in fact, less, partly because the blood vessels have narrowed, bringing less blood, and partly because carbon monoxide from the cigarette smoke has actually depleted the blood's ability to carry oxygen. Carbon monoxide combines more readily with haemoglobin than oxygen, which is why people can commit suicide by running their car engines in an enclosed space. Exhausts give off carbon monoxide.

Smokers believe that in the short term cigarettes help them to get through the day. They are well aware of the long-term bad effects, but they genuinely believe that the short-term effects are good for them. This is not true: the addiction is confusing them, quite genuinely. The signals are being crossed at a subconscious level. Nobody is to blame. The belief, or the sensation prompting the belief, is genuine.

Let us take a look at the short-term bad effects of cigarette smoking before moving on to understanding and tackling the tricks of the addiction. Here they are:

● When inhaling cigarette smoke the lethal gas carbon monoxide is inhaled as well, at levels some 600 times above the safe levels set in industry.

● 4,000 other chemicals, many of them poisonous, are also inhaled, including hydrogen cyanide, carbolic acid and arsenic trioxide.

● Nicotine itself is also a deadly poison; in fact if the nicotine in one pack of cigarettes were to be injected into a smoker it would kill them. That is why the heart pounds, to try and evict the poisons quickly.

TACKLING THE ADDICTION

Smokers are usually interesting people. They are people who have had to fight against adversity, come up from the ranks or battle against authority figures. They are not going to let anybody tell them how to live their lives – which is laudable. The problem is that somewhere along the line, while they developed their individuality and their right to live life as they see fit, the habit of smoking got tacked on to some of the actions by which they arrived at their freedom (e.g. rebellions against unfair or restrictive authority).

The addiction has attached itself to the memory, but the memory has long since subsided into the subconscious. Thus, a teenager who has been repeatedly told by parents not to smoke will not recall when he or she is an adult that this was one of the ways of defying parental authority, so that every time they light a cigarette they are in fact reinforcing that right to be an individual.

Smokers are rebels, and rebels make the world go round. But regrettably they have got their individuality hooked onto a very destructive habit.

BREAKING THE ADDICTION

Many of the stop-smoking techniques work on aversion, on repressing the desire to smoke. This is like trying to repress a volcano; it will only break out in another place, and that is why smokers who give up often feel deprived or depressed or take to food or suffer loss of sleep or find they cannot concentrate. The repression technique is not repressing the desire to smoke so much as repressing the very spirit of the person, which has become tied to the desire to smoke.

Acknowledging and understanding the underlying link with their past bid for identity is the first step to giving up, because it then becomes possible to see the desire to smoke for what it is and to detach it from its other mental connotations.

Physical addiction to smoking is easy to give up: this is why smokers can give up for some time, only to be prompted to start again by some little thing. Mental addiction is what has to be recognized and tackled.

ON TOP OF OLD SMOKEY: GIVING UP SURVIVAL KIT
Here are some suggestions for smokers wanting to give up for good:

1. Never tell anyone you are giving up – rewards and pats on the back for doing so will make you feel trapped if you start again. Attention is the last thing you need.
2. Never say never again. You will never lose the desire to smoke, although it will occur less and less. Recognize the desire, don't repress it. It will only last about 30 seconds.
3. Don't substitute smoking for another bad habit. This will only misdirect the addiction onto something else, such as eating, which will mean that it will simply take longer to get to grips with the addiction. That said, you could allow yourself two weeks' grace while you have a stack of crudités in the fridge in order to nibble on a carrot stick, if desperate, or chew gum – but never let it go on for longer than the initial period of grace.
4. Accept that you are a smoker who is stopped for now. Never tell anyone you're given up for good (people love to tempt providence).
5. Acknowledge your desire to smoke as and when it happens – don't repress it. Recognize that it is attached to a series of steps you took in your past on the way to becoming you. Now you have other options to tie that to.
6. Keep to your daily and social routines – don't shy away from places where you know you will want to smoke, or you will only make yourself more aware that you want to smoke.

PHYSICAL EFFECTS OF GIVING UP
For a few weeks you will feel worse. Your body has adjusted to your habit of smoking and will react when deprived of it. Symptoms that have been suppressed may resurface, for example running sinuses, coughing, wheezing, a bad taste in the mouth, or tingly extremities. This is the body going through the reverse process of what happened when you started smoking. Think of it as the body getting its own back for a bit, while normalizing its circuits.

Feeling light-headed, dizzy or disorientated is caused simply because you are now getting more oxygen than you are used to. This will settle down after a day or two, and you will feel more mentally alert than before.

Difficulty getting to sleep is often a complex chain of effects. Smokers are usually coffee drinkers, and it may be that the caffeine you are drinking is affecting you more, now that it is not competing with nicotine for absorption in your blood. In any case, drink decaffeinated coffee until the worst effects are over. After that it will be necessary to give up that as well, because it contains two other stimulants that are not removed in the decaffeination process as well as the chemical by-products of the process itself! Note also that cola drinks, tea, some pre menstrual tension remedies and many pain killers contain caffeine.

Constipation is noticed by many people who give up smoking. Nicotine does stimulate the bowel. It may be necessary to take two table-spoonsful of psyllium husks in a glass of fruit juice daily to combat this, or some other herbal bowel stimulant.

Accept that any advice such as the above can only help. You have to find your own way. There are smokers who have given up for love, after aversion therapy, after hypnosis, after falling off a cliff (if they're still alive), after every conceivable incident. That doesn't mean it will work that way for you – or for your friend who wants to give up.

The consensus of opinion/advice above was largely gleaned from one of the most experienced experts ever to have given up smoking herself. For more than 10 years she examined the comparative success rates of every giving-up technique from the standpoint of the permanence of their success rate. She is an American called Gillian Riley, and her entire post-smoking life has been directed towards helping others to quit. She gives courses in London (see Useful Addresses) and has written a book, *How to Stop Smoking and Stay Stopped for Good*.

The book, excellent though it is, is no substitute for her courses and for the year's telephone help-line she provides afterwards.

HYPERVENTILATION – OVERBREATHING

Look back and re-read the first few paragraphs of this chapter. This was a test to establish whether you were an overbreather or not. Quite apart from affecting the vital balance of oxygen and carbon dioxide in the blood, overbreathing is just as bad in its own way as smoking, since both habits induce the body to remain on a kind of red alert. The body soon learns to tone this down to a pink alert, otherwise it would exhaust itself, but this in turn means that no genuine stress can be met with full power, neither can the body really relax. It is a bit like revving a car with the gear in neutral – there is a lot of smoke but you get nowhere fast, and you soon deplete your fuel and burn out your engine.

Thoracic (chest) breathing is known to be associated with stress-induced illnesses and conditions such as high blood pressure, coronary disease, high cholesterol levels and irritable bowel syndrome, quite apart from lowering the amount of oxygen that gets to the brain (through altering the normal carbon dioxide/oxygen ratio). One medical study showed that 30 per cent of patients with high blood pressure could come off their tablets just by practising to breathe diaphragmatically; another 30 per cent could have their tablets reduced.

To understand why this is so, it is necessary to look at what each type of breathing means to the body. The automatic nervous system of the body, which regulates heartbeat, temperature, activities of the bowel and so forth, has two branches, the sympathetic and the parasympathetic. One governs the arousal response and one governs the corresponding relaxation response. Thoracic, or chest breathing, is known to be related to the arousal response, since during arousal we need to get air fast into the lungs, for flight or fight. And so we raise our shoulders and expand our chests, getting quick breaths into the lungs. The sharp intake of breath when shocked is an example of this arousal response.

Parasympathetic activity occurs when the crisis is over and we can relax. Then we sigh, letting air out of the lungs, take one or two deep breaths from the pit of our stomachs and 'breathe again' – literally. Or so it should be. The problem is that the learned response of thoracic breathing sometimes dominates our waking hours, triggered perhaps by a vigorous exercise breathing pattern being carried over into daily life, or by a long-forgotten shock (still holding our breaths), or by restrictive clothing to keep the stomach in (women do this for appearance's sake but men's belts can be just as bad.

The result is that a breathing pattern associated with challenge by the body is not reserved for when it is needed but maintained all the time.

RE-LEARNING TO BREATHE; POSITIVE ADVANTAGES
Fortunately, it is not difficult to learn to re-breathe, and the advantages will be many, since a relaxation technique will be learned at the same time.

Breathing is a virtually unique body process in that it can take place without our thinking about it, and also we can alter it at will. As such, it is a vital link between the conscious part of our being and the automatic or unconscious part. Stored in the unconscious part are all the traumas and forgotten memories of the past that have conspired over the years to make us permanently tense, to react like Pavlov's dogs to situations that, as mature adults, we could handle easily.

By redirecting the breathing and focusing the attention on the breath (and not the thoughts) we can, in a matter of minutes, learn to relax.

Here is how: choose a quiet place where you are alone when you start. Take off any restrictive clothing, including footwear, and lie down where you can stretch out completely. Cover yourself with a blanket if you feel you will be cold. Lie on your back and after a minute or so of normal breathing place your left hand on your chest and your right on a spot over and just below your navel. Be aware of which hand is moving more as you breathe. After a minute or so gently follow your natural exhalation by pressing down on your stomach with your right hand. Release the pressure and let your air intake gently push your right hand up. Let your chest relax; don't tense it while doing this.

After a while you will capture the feeling of this new rhythm.

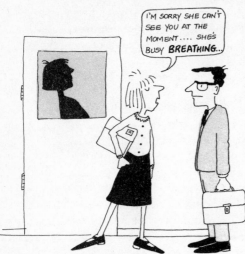

Now you are ready for the next stage, which is akin to meditation. As you breathe in and out, do so to the count of 4; inhale ... two, three, four, exhale ... two, three, four. Try to smooth any jerks or pauses in your breathing so that the inhalation and exhalation flow smoothly into each other.

If any thoughts arise, let them float away. Don't try to block them out, acknowledge them. Tell yourself that you will think about them later, and return your concentration to your breathing. Carry on counting your breathing rhythm.

Ten minutes of this when you return home from work, or a conscious re-direction of your breathing when you are sitting in a traffic jam, unable to sleep, late for an appointment, or worried about a loved one, will help you to conserve your adrenalin and lower your stress level.

One young surgeon was noted to be very much more lively at the end of a day of operating than her colleagues. When asked about it she said: 'I keep reminding myself to breathe deeply during my day.' That simple technique enabled her to get through the day in better shape than her colleagues.

For those who find trying to breathe correctly is almost more stressful than breathing their normal way, just deepening the breath and slowing its pace consciously can effect the transition from one type of breathing to another.

You believe that all you are doing is directing your attention to your breathing rhythm, but in fact your body is responding through its unconscious circuits to your focus. It is not important how something happens, so long as it happens. There is a tape available to help you learn to breathe more effectively (see Useful Addresses).

7

*

THE NERVOUS SYSTEM AND BRAIN

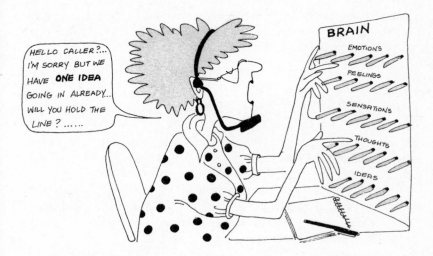

IN THIS CHAPTER

✻ Brain power ✻ Mystery of consciousness ✻ How nerves
work ✻ The body electric ✻ Understanding reflexes
✻ Parental conditioning and its hidden effects ✻ Stress and
sussing your stressors ✻ Anti-stress techniques/therapies
✻ The tranquillizer trap ✻ Decoding and defusing depression
✻ Nervous breakdown ✻ Children, drugs and diet (new ways
of protecting them) ✻ And finally to sleep . . .

The saying 'I think, therefore I am' has become part and parcel of our culture. We – that is, our consciousness – reside in our brains. An individual may lose almost any other part of his body – a kidney, a limb, half a liver, or indeed, as transplants have shown, exchange his heart for another without losing identity. His brain, however, seems to be 'where he lives'.

The brain and the nervous system control nearly everything that goes on in the body. Like the wiring in a car or the electricity in a house, nothing works without it.

Because of the supremacy of our brain power, we, *Homo sapiens*, rule the world. Even the most ordinary person can prevail over the animal and plant kingdom on Earth. But such supremacy hasn't happened overnight, and the story is really riveting. Millions of years of evolutionary trial and error have enabled us to adapt to our environment in a way that has led to the orchestration of modern life and civilization as we know it. Little wonder that the brain and nervous system are the most complex of the body's systems.

HOW BRAINPOWER BEGINS

As little as 18 days after the fertilization of a human egg, the brain starts to develop, and by three months (a mere 12 weeks of pregnancy) its basic outlines are formed. The development is both fast and fantastic, so that by the time the infant is two years old, its brain structure is virtually the same as that of an adult. No wonder the heads of infants are so disproportionately large compared with the rest of their bodies – the brain is indeed what develops first and fastest and what dominates life.

In fact, the birth moment can be seen to arrive just in time, while the infant is not so helpless that it cannot survive, but yet still has a small enough head to pass through the mother's pelvis. Already, the brain will weigh about 350g (12oz); by two years old that will have increased to 1,000g (2.2lb). It grows a mere 300g (10oz) after that, in order to arrive at its adult size, which it reaches by puberty.

The rapid maturation of the brain makes the first two years of life crucial. Although we are born with as many neurons (brain cells) as we will ever have (about 10,000 million in the brain cortex alone) if there is insufficient protein in the infant's diet during these crucial early years (ideally derived from protein-rich breast milk and later from food), the infant may be retarded. The intelligence of many hundreds of millions of the world's potentially normal children may continue to be impaired as long as so many of them – 60 per cent is the current estimate – suffer from inadequate diets. And not all these children live in

Third World countries; many of them are alive and unwell in Britain and other Western countries today (see Children, Diet and Stress, later in this chapter and read about diet in Chapter 4).

The above is a little known but vital fact about the potential of human intelligence. Better known are the somewhat disconcerting facts that we all lose about 50,000 brain cells a day between the ages of 20 and 70, resulting in one-tenth less brain power when we are old. But this is balanced by the mysterious estimate that we use only one-tenth of our brain anyway throughout life. There are more mysteries associated with the brain and brain power than any other area of the body.

THE MYSTERY OF CONSCIOUSNESS

In fact, one of these mysteries is worth mentioning now, one that has been puzzling scientists and neurologists ever since they started examining the brain, and that is: where **does** consciousness reside? Experiments have shown that as much as 50 per cent of the brain can be destroyed in any area, and yet memory still exists of what has gone on in the life.

Incredibly, modern scientific belief now contends that the mind is a separate entity from the brain and possibly interacts with the brain in much the same way as a computer program interacts with – drives – a computer, the mind being the program (software) and the brain being the computer (hardware). In other words, the mind controls the brain in much the same way as an architect's blueprint controls the design of a house.

However, much is still to be discovered. What is unusual is that scientists actually admit that there are whole areas of brain/mind function about which they know very little.

Nonetheless, the basic structure of the brain and central nervous system is known, and it helps to understand at least the rudiments of this, because behind these workings exists the real key to to one of the major health threats of the 20th century – stress, the underlying cause of most disease. There is barely a person alive who has avoided the sapping effects of this contemporary condition, whose origins are perceived deep within the brain and nervous system.

HOW AND WHY NERVES WORK

The nervous system, which includes the brain, is a system of many parts, reaching to the remotest boundaries of the body. Anyone who has ever had a nerve cut or suffered that most exquisite of nerve discomforts that a certain type of blow to the elbow can cause, knows that all feeling, all communication within the body, whether painful or pleasurable, comes through the nerve supply.

In fact the whole purpose of the nervous system is to coordinate and respond to the environment, to create a communication system through which information may be passed and motivation for the appropriate activity given.

NERVES ON AUTO

As with a telephone system, the nervous system is a two-way system, inflow and outflow, and functionally it is further divided into those parts of it that are under the control of our consciousness (manually controlled) and those parts that are not (automatic), i.e. the voluntary and involuntary parts. It is the involuntary part of it, otherwise known as the autonomic nervous system, which has been the recipient of so much medical attention in recent years, because of its association with stress.

THE NATURE OF NERVES

The nerve cells of the nervous system are called neurones, and they make up the basic structural and functional unit of the circuits and networks of the human nervous system.

Nerves may be grey or white, depending on whether they have a myelin (fatty) sheath, as larger nerves tend to have, or not, in which case they are grey. Two things must strike 'familiar' chords here: the word 'myelin', which occurs in the descriptions of certain nervous diseases such as poliomyelitis, and the grey and white appearance of nerves, as may be seen in any brain tissue.

Only in remote parts of the body are solitary nerves seen; they more usually occur in bundles, and most of them travel to their body sites in cables enclosed by a protective fibrous sheath, which for all the world resemble co-axial cable! The similarity is further emphasized when it is seen that nerves carry a charge and that their impulses communicate by means of a very delicate and extremely weak type of electricity.

THE BODY ELECTRIC

The way in which electricity is generated in the body is an anatomical and chemical wonder, too complex to enter into in a book of this kind. Suffice it to say that the necessary charge is developed by an interplay between sodium and potassium ions (ions are extremely tiny particles smaller than molecules), and thus the balance of sodium and potassium in the body is of prime importance to healthy nerve functioning. This points directly to another health factor of great significance, for in today's diet the intake of sodium in the form of common salt is often so great as to threaten to interfere with this basic body process. Salt exists in the modern diet not only in overt forms, such as salt on the table and in cooking, but in hidden forms such as in the fat in sausages, hamburgers, cold meats, tinned foods, smoked and preserved foods and so on. Potassium is much harder to come by and is mainly found in leafy green vegetables and fruits such as apricots and bananas. We have collectively become a nation of salt-eaters, or as some might say, well-preserved in brine, with the resultant insidious effect on our nervous systems.

Furthermore, we do not exercise as did our forefathers, whose work was more manual and who were, therefore, more able to sweat off any excess salt they ate.

THE IMPORTANCE OF NERVES

A nerve lost is often lost forever. For although nerve regeneration can occur in the body, it is slow and does not happen invariably. This is known by any one who has actually suffered nerve damage through a deep cut or operation wound: there is always a numb spot on the wound. This of course is the extreme, but think of a case in which the nerves are simply not functioning as well as they could in a body, when they are irritable, sluggish, struggling against chemical imbalances, in other words **on edge** . . . ring any bells?

Most people are aware that it is nerves and nerve impulses that cause the muscles in the body to contract and hence move according to our desires. This is the truest of the voluntary nervous system, in which the effects are more obvious because they are under conscious control, but it is also more subtly true of that part of the nervous system (involuntary) that is not under our conscious control. What is unshakeable is that nothing moves, nothing happens in the body without the healthy functioning of the nervous system. The sad sight of a paraplegic – a person who has suffered injury or disease to the central nervous system – makes us all too aware of this fact. Serious injuries to the spinal cord cut off both movement and sensation, the two major nerve functions, below the injury site and they do so forever.

Nervous diseases can do the same. They have been brought more to our attention in recent years by such courageous and inspiring cases as that of the brilliant scientist, Stephen Hawking, who has one of these diseases.

FIRING NERVES!

What happens when a nerve fires, or is activated by an impulse from the brain, is a fascinating sequence of events, which depends not only on the electrical activity of the nerves but also on chemical activity, since chemicals are needed to create links as well.

The structural unit of the nervous system, the neuron, has evolved to do this delicate task over millions of years of evolution, and its whole purpose is to enable the organism to respond to its environment in the best possible way for further survival. Thus the basic function of the nerve cell reflects this principle. A stimulus, such as standing on a tack, occurs, the nerves in the foot become aware of the stimulus and alert the brain, which responds with an order to lift the foot – fast! Stimulus → awareness → response → reflex action.

In that simple sequence lies the complex structure of life as we live it. But it is the increasing complexity of life that is causing the challenge, the stress to us.

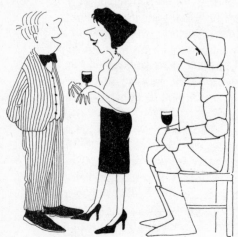

OUR **UNCONSCIOUSLY CONDITIONED ARMOUR** MAY BE AFFECTING THE QUALITY OF OUR LIVES......

CONDITIONED REFLEX

This is because reflexes can be modified by learning and by conditioning. For example, every driver knows the reflex action of putting your foot where the brake would be when being driven by another driver who (in your opinion) hasn't braked soon enough! The reflex in this case has become unconscious – a part of our unconscious armouring against life and its dangers, learned from past experiences, in this case in traffic. Some would say in the traffic of life.

An example of such reflexes and how they become part of our unconscious armouring occurred when a scientist called Pavlov trained dogs. When he fed them he also rang a bell. After a while he just had to ring the bell for the dogs to start salivating.

PARENTAL CONDITIONING

Parents and elders can condition us, well or badly, wittingly or unwittingly, to respond in certain ways to stimuli, which may give rise to a pattern being formed that is not appropriate for adult life nor very healthy either.

Luckily, there are ways to unlearn such responses or certainly to monitor and control them (see below), but first we need to understand them and know about them through the medium of understanding the nervous system, and in particular those parts of it that are responsible for those reflexes that have become part of our unconsciously conditioned armour. They may be affecting the quality of our lives and, by casting a blight over some organic function such as heart function or digestion, endangering health itself.

THE BODY ON AUTO

The most important aspect of the nervous system, from the ordinary person's point of view, is the autonomic nervous system, so called because it functions regardless of whether we are concentrating on it or not – autonomic = automatic. Like everything in life it is not as simple as that, because we can affect the autonomic function by our thoughts and emotions.

The autonomic system has two branches, the sympathetic and the parasympathetic. Both of them are concerned with keeping us on the road of life or, as the doctors might say, they help to keep the body's internal environment constant. To do this they maintain temperature, fluid balance and blood consistency. They also control some vital body processes, such as heart rate, digestion and respiration. All smooth muscles, not only those in blood vessels but also those in the glands, are under their control.

SOS RESPONSES

The sympathetic branch of the autonomic nervous system is responsible for what we know as the fight or flight response. Basically it enables the body to handle emergencies or sudden environmental changes. This autonomic function of the nervous system has been around for millions of years, virtually unchanged, and thus it dates back to the time when our ancestors were covered with hair. The so-called fight or flight mechanism evolved to aid our predecessors to turn and fight or to run like mad in the face of danger or a challenge, such as meeting a tiger head on!

The actual automatic nervous responses can be better understood with this in mind. To this day they involve increases in heartbeat and breathing rates, muscles being tensed (ready for running or fighting) and, because all these activities threaten to overheat the body, the hands and feet becoming familiarly clammy (the rest of the body was covered in fur, all those ages ago, so these were the obvious hairless parts on which to concentrate the cooling mechanism). Digestion is stopped, as an activity which can be continued later when the stress or danger has passed (hence the mouth goes dry – no saliva) and the body is, in fact, aroused for a bout of frantic activity.

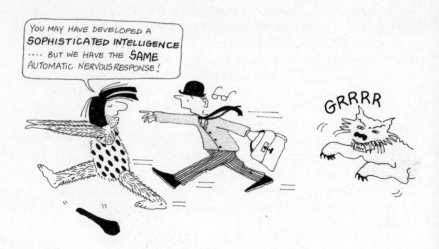

This picture is just as familiar today – on the shop floor, in the office or in a traffic jam, at an airport or in an exam or at home during a family argument – as it was then. The only problem is we don't usually run like mad any more, and we don't usually fight off an enemy physically. Thus the energy generated, instead of being dissipated by physical activity, gets stored in the body systems, overloading them as surely as three or four plugs from the one electrical socket will overload a power point. That is what we now call stress.

RELAXATION RESPONSE

The corresponding relaxation response is designed to come into play once the stress has been removed. We sigh, letting out the breath we have been holding in our lungs, our muscles relax, very often we hear our stomach begin to gurgle (signifying the reinstating of the digestive process), our pulse rate drops, and we take a nap or a rest until we feel strong again. The parasympathetic branch of the autonomic nervous system, involving the relaxation response, is designed to conserve body energy and return the body to the *status quo* of normal functioning. (The parasympathetic system produces body energy, the sympathetic uses it.)

What goes wrong, of course, is that we don't now live in caveman conditions, though we do have caveman emotions (these also are very old).

WHAT CAUSES STRESS?

Among the conditions that can cause stress now as they did then are pain, rage, fright, cold and overwork and to those we must now include the many drugs and medications we take. We must also include the lifestyles lead, chained to desks or VDUs (themselves stressful), waiting in queues for family assistance, sitting in traffic jams, and worst of all, dealing with crises and with family relationships. It has been said that 'there is no auto-nomic activity that cannot be modified, even completely disorganized, by emotional upsets'. One classic example of how the nervous system reacts to an emotion, in this case embarrassment, is seen in blushing. This involves a rapid change in the distribution of the body's blood supply; later in life that could lead to a more wide-spread response that would be bad for blood pressure. We are also familiar with the opposite effect – that is of going white, as blood drains from the face and extremities in response to a 'fear' situation such as stage fright or before tests, interviews or examina-tions. Such reactions, themselves nat-ural and harmless responses to the environment, may be augmented by the pressures of modern life, and, if they are not addressed, they can lead to the system being permanently under stress. Fright, anger or appre-hension can completely upset digest-ive processes and at the same time may cause blood pressure to rise and

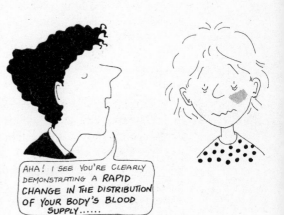

heartrate to increase. If any of these emotions becomes stored in the body because of repeated reinforcement, such as being close to someone who habitually makes you angry, the balancing relaxation response can be rendered ineffectual.

The need for physical exercise to work off stress can be seen in this context to be vital, as it replaces the activity that burned off stress all those millions of years ago in fighting or fleeing.

Fortunately for the lounge lizards, there are other ways of dealing with stress besides exercise. Indeed, learning one or other of the techniques mentioned later in this chapter could be quite literally a lifesaving meas-ure for all those in stressful situations, including those who exercise, since not all forms of modern stress are addressed by exercise as once they were. Our ancestors did not have to deal with tax, social security, mortgages, mothers-in-law (well, perhaps they fought them!), traffic jams, working cheek by jowl in offices or factories, commuting, divorces or any of the million stressful features of contemporary life. True, they had to deal with tigers and other wild animals, but paper tigers are much, much worse. Stress is something we must all get to grips with, partly by adopting techniques that support the relaxation response and partly by changing mind-sets.

STRESS AND BODY SYSTEMS; PSYCHONEUROIMMUNOLOGY

It has now been scientifically proved that the way we think – whether positively or negatively, happily or unhappily – can actually affect our physical health. Through the limbic system, which is a very old part of the brain that controls automatic body functioning, worry and stress generated from the brain's more recently evolved 'thinking' centres are directly passed to various organs of the body. Which organs are affected depends on individual factors such as personal experience influencing conditioned reflexes, inherited weaknesses and so on. We can no longer deny that wittingly or unwittingly we are directly responsible for our illnesses and that they are an expression of our lives.

Far from being a distressing fact, this is one of the most reassuring aspects of modern health knowledge: that which we have done, we can undo. It may take a little longer to untie the knot that it did to tie it, for as any sailor knows, knots tend to get stuck, but untying, as long as we know the process, is possible. As Louise Hay said in her now-famous book of the same title: 'You can heal your life.'

ASSESSING YOUR PERSONAL STRESS LEVEL

Because stress seems to be the common factor underlying most diseases, let us look at what stress is and how to deal with it. Here are some points to consider, but before reading on, jot down what you think is causing stress in your own life today. Write down the causes in the space provided. Don't feel guilty at laying stress at the door of your family: it gives them the freedom to do the same!

Now compare your stress triggers with those most commonly experienced by society. *Note:* The following list is very often printed in books and magazines accompanied by a scale of values from which you score – death of a spouse being top of the list and stressors such as minor violations of the law being at the bottom: but there is a school of thought, to which I subscribe, which believes that what stresses one person leaves another untouched – sometimes death of a spouse is a relief! Sometimes a minor violation of the law can lead to a heart attack – so no particular values are given here.

1. Problems or changes affecting relationships within the family circle. These include serious marital problems, changes in children and their lives, including their leaving home – or just arriving!
2. Sex and other marital problems (sleeping with the enemy!)
3. Changes in the number of arguments had or provoked
4. Changes at work, including being fired or hired or changes in the hierarchy
5. Prison terms or brushes with the law or other major authorities such as the Inland Revenue
6. Mortgage and other financial problems; poor housing conditions, including dependent relatives living at home
7. Move of home and/or district or country
8. Serious changes in health of self or other family member
9. Not sleeping (which is really a symptom of another stress factor)
10. Revision of personal habits, such as starting a diet
11. Outstanding personal achievement or love affair (or somebody else's achievement or love affair!)
12. Problems with friends/social life/loneliness
13. Holidays, birthdays and Christmas (either so good you feel let down afterwards or so bad you feel let down afterwards)
14. And, of course, the death of someone dear to you including a pet.

You could give yourself a score if you like, so many points for so many factors, but since that might be stressful, perhaps it would be more useful to examine how stressed you may be by alternative means.
    Consider the following signs of stress:

1. Needing a drink/cigarette/pill
2. Migraine
3. High blood pressure and palpitations
4. Anxiety (especially if you can't put your finger on its cause)
5. Neck and other muscle tensions
6. Menstrual problems, sexual problems, including impotence
7. Indigestion
8. Depression
9. Irritability, including talking to yourself
10. Drinking or eating food quickly
11. Biting your nails or lips, tapping your feet or fingers, clearing your throat, constant swallowing or any other nervous habit
12. Impatient to finish other people's sentences

13. Lying awake worrying
14. Walking, driving and so on in a perpetual hurry
15. Mislaying things
16. Looking around for something to do all the time – feeling guilty about resting
17. Getting aggressive with animate and inanimate objects when they get in your way
18. Sensitivity to noise
19. Neglecting your dress/appearance
20. Sweating, flushing and other rapid temperature changes
21. Reading lists of stress symptoms!

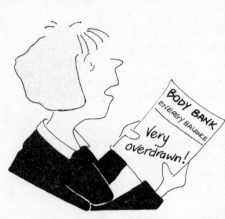

Enough of lists – the time has come to discover just how easy it is to understand and deal with stress. It is not really important to identify what stress you have, although of course that helps. Just as it helps to use the right club in golf, or the right stain-remover to take out a stain.

EFFECTS OF STRESS

As we have seen, stress puts the body into the fight or flight mode, which means that respiration increases, heart rate does likewise, digestion stops (which is why it is unwise to eat when stressed, as the food simply hangs around in the digestive system putrefying, just as it would on a win-dowsill on a hot day), blood supply to other vital organs is side-tracked to the muscles, which, if we do not then use them to fight or flee, means we tense them.

This is soon followed by tiredness, the body's way of protecting itself – it can't always be on red alert – and thus anyone who feels more or less perpetually tired need look no further to know that they are stressed. Stress uses up the valuable body-bank of energy, and unless it is compensated for by the corresponding relaxation response, which conserves and preserves energy, will quickly lead to exhaustion. One thing must be understood and that is this: it is possible to have an overdraft situation in the body just as it is at the bank. Let this go on for too long and the body calls in the overdraft by getting sick – the only way it knows to guarantee it a rest so it can get on with repairing some of its tissues. That is why frequent colds, allergies and other common infections are often signs of stress.

In order to get the body into the relaxation mode, which over years of rushing we have persuaded it to shelve, we have to learn to become aware of our own stress symptoms. Or we can simply assume, as some people do, that we are stressed and take measures to control it without bothering to find out the details. That is why many people learn to meditate – whatever and wherever the stress, it will be helped by this technique, if it is practised regularly.

ANTI-STRESS MEASURES

Here are a variety of techniques that are known and proved to alleviate symptoms of stress.

BIOFEEDBACK
This is a most interesting technique and one that is quickly learned, but you must initially go to class to do so (very entertaining because there are a lot of other people there in the same leaky boat as you). Basically it enables you to become aware of your specific stress area by externalizing signs of it on a very simple meter loosely strapped to the hand – a stress meter!

Once the meter level is there under your watchful eye, you can monitor your stress level and see what arouses it. You can then learn and practise a variety of relaxation techniques to lower the meter level and hence your stress, again monitoring the results. This is not 'hit and miss'.

Through biofeedback, people with debilitating and sometimes dangerous stress symptoms have transformed their lives. For example, sufferers from stress headaches can learn in a few lessons how to relax their forehead muscles and hence arrest the process by which the headache takes hold. Those who suffer from high blood pressure can learn to recognize the situations that increase it and then to practise a technique that lowers it. It is possible, through learning in this way, to control stomach acidity and temperature of extremities, which is useful in cases of severely impaired circulation, such as with Reynaud's disease.

Biofeedback in itself does not deal with the stress, it only teaches you how to recognize and measure it. Similarly the bathroom scales will tell you if you are overweight, but not how to lose it! Hence biofeedback is nearly always taught in conjunction with relaxation techniques: one without the other is pointless.

Some may argue that it seems unnecessary to learn the biofeedback technique if it is the relaxation technique that matters, but biofeedback is useful in certain instances for two reasons. First, in order to control stress, some people have to know when it is happening and how, since reaction to stress is often unconscious. Second, relaxation techniques and their efficacy vary from person to person; with biofeedback several can be tried and the best one chosen. Men in particular seem to relate well to the biofeedback technique. Possibly this is because men have always liked to peer into the works, to see what is happening, then to learn to control it, whereas women are more likely to accept that it is happening and to be prepared to move on to the relaxation concept. Women live more in the world of feelings than men, and consequently they know their bodies better.

MEDITATION

This type of relaxation technique works particularly well for those who are prepared to discipline themselves to sit down quietly for 15 minutes every morning and evening and practise a form of meditation. This can be an extremely simple process involving cycles of counting the breaths while breathing in and out deeply from the pit of the stomach, or it can involve learning a mantra, a word that is repeated over and over during the meditation. There is nothing occult or dangerous about this, the word is used simply to stop the brain from thinking about other words, such as overdraft, workload, health, shopping list or missing item.

Meditation is a technique which applies itself to all forms of stress, whatever body area is affected. It is of particular value in hyperventilation (overbreathing), which is an extremely common and potentially damaging stress symptom very common in men (See Chapter 6).

The mantra type of meditation technique is taught particularly successfully by the Transcendental Meditation Group, which is now worldwide, with teaching centres in most cities. People think of TM, as it is now called, as having religious connotations, but in fact nobody is required to alter their beliefs in order to learn TM. More than 600 clinical studies have absolutely proved its efficacy in controlling stress.

Learning TM is remarkably simple and takes about four lessons of an hour's duration, plus one or two checks at later intervals. Look them up in the telephone book or see Useful Addresses.

EXERCISE, MASSAGE AND OTHER DE-STRESSORS

Vigorous exercise, even competitive exercise, is wonderful for taking one's mind off one's stress. In replacing one form of stress with another, it completely relaxes that part of the mind that was absorbed with the regular stressors of life. Also, the body gets a chance to express in a natural way the flight or fight response and after it the equally natural relaxation response. Consider exercise as one vital part of an anti-stress programme. It doesn't matter what kind of exercise you choose – dancing, yoga, aerobics – all can work well, but don't overlook the simplest of all exercises, walking. Brisk walking is both good exercise and a process that aids clear thinking. So walk and you may solve the problems that are on your mind.

Additional techniques, which work better for some than others, include humour – watching funny movies on video, for example. Research has shown that laughter actually releases calming hormones into the bloodstream.

Any form of water therapy is soothing, from swimming to simply taking a warm bath. And massage is also helpful. Two techniques you should seriously consider are foot massage (see the section on reflexology in Chapter 8) and aromatherapy, which concentrates on the entire neuro-muscular system (see Chapter 11).

Self-massage is another beneficial avenue to explore. There is an excellent book by Jaqueline Young, *Self Massage*, which instructs in the finding and massage of key pressure points in the body for the purposes of achieving relief from many different forms of stress.

STRESSORS: THE ANTAGONISTS OF RELAXATION

On the other side of the balance sheet are the stressors. In addition to the mental and emotional factors previously discussed, it may be surprising to learn that things we sometimes do and take to relieve stress are, in fact, adding to it. For example, drinking tea, coffee, cola or other caffeine-containing liquids is not relaxing at all. Caffeine stimulates the body to perform in the fight or flight mode. So try the herb teas and drinks that are available instead or take guarana (see Useful Addresses, Rio Trading), which will lift your spirits without eliciting as many side-effects as caffeine would.

SMOKING
Having a cigarette is not relaxing either. Nicotine is a stressor. Read how smoking actually drains your nervous energy, while making you believe it is doing the reverse, in Chapter 6.

A WORD ABOUT DRINKING AND STRESS
Alcohol can actually defuse stress, provided it is taken in moderation. One or two drinks at the end of the day have been shown to be relaxing, especially if they are taken with a friend, since 'having a moan' is another way of defusing stress. Any more than two drinks, however, and alcohol becomes a stressor, interfering with sleep rhythms (even if you stay asleep) and causing depression.

DRUGS AND TRANQUILLIZERS; A NEGATIVE VIEW OF THE TRANQUILLIZER TRAP

Drugs and tranquillizers, including sleeping pills, do not apply themselves to the basic cause of stress, except in its acute stage. At best they simply control the symptoms. Look at it another way: aspirin does not cure headaches, it merely controls the symptom – the headache – which will recur under the same conditions another time unless the cause is addressed.

In addition, the taking of tranquillizers and sleeping pills to control, not cure, stress quickly becomes addictive, sometimes in a matter of two to four weeks, which in itself is stressful!

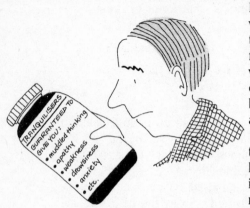

Also these chemicals – because that is what they are – take longer to leave the body than the few hours in which they take effect on the condition. Hence the person is always fighting the drug, in much the same way as one contends with a hangover. At best these remedies should be used in the short term to deal with a crisis, not as a long-term prop.

Another good reason for confining their use to the short term is the little known fact that they are only effective in controlling the symptom for a maximum of four weeks. This is why many people say they have the best night's sleep for years when they start taking tranquillizers or sleeping pills, but after a while their effectiveness wears off.

Here are a few more points not found on the manufacturer's labels:

Tranquillizers and sleeping pills contain what is essentially the same substance – Benzodiazepine – and Valium, Ativan, Mogadon and Dalmane are very similar. Why is it, then, that some are marketed as sleeping tablets and others as tranquillizers? Because they sell more that way – you have to buy two items instead of one. The tranquillizer business is multi-billion.

Just consider these statistics relating to Britain: 14 per cent of the adult population currently uses them; 5 million people take them every night to sleep; 3 million people have used them for a protracted time (at least six months); 25 million prescriptions are written every year for them in their various uses – for sleep and tranquillizing. Similar figures exist in most western countries. No wonder the US

Drug Abuse Warning Network announced as long ago as 1980 that the popular tranquillizer Valium was the most abused of all drugs, and that includes heroin.

And that is not all: it would appear that once the widespread use of tranquillizers was recognized and prescriptions for them began to fall in the late 80s, there was a corresponding rise in the prescribing of beta blockers. In the late 80s (no official figures were available at the time of going to press) this amounted to nearly 15 million prescriptions – 23 per cent of all drugs prescribed (source: MIND Information).

Here are a few more facts, namely a list of their side-effects:

● Muddled thinking

● The 'couldn't care less' feeling

● Weakness and lack of muscular coordination

● Drowsiness

● Low blood pressure (which can be as undesirable as high blood pressure)

● Anxiety

● Insomnia

● Hypersensitivity to light and sound

● Shaking, sweating

● Visual disturbances

● Palpitations

● Loss of memory

● Difficulty doing skilled work

And ... wait for it ... **depression**, the very state for which the tablets are often prescribed.

Let's be reasonable, however; tranquillizers do have positive benefits.

HOW/WHEN TO USE TRANQUILLIZERS: A POSITIVE VIEW
First, people suffering from shock or bereavement or a similar circumstance can be helped to get over the initial trauma with tranquillizers. Second, people with serious mental disorders, rather than the disturbances for which most of us take tranquillizers, can be enabled to function in the community and to lead worthwhile lives when their sometimes serious symptoms are controlled. In this case the powerful tranquillizers they are given are addressing mental illness, and although they still have side effects, these are more than outweighed by the ter-

rible symptoms from which they would otherwise suffer – people with schizophrenia, for example, sometimes hear voices telling them how to think or what to do.

KICKING THE TRANQUILLIZER HABIT

Coming off tranquillizers can be a long and arduous procedure. However, there are many help-groups, such as MIND and TRANX RELEASE in Britain, both of which have regional branches. There is also a tape you can send for (see Useful Addresses under BHMA)

First you should tell your family practitioner that you want to start withdrawing and enlist aid. If he or she is unhelpful or insists on your continuing, do at least get another opinion, preferably from another doctor outside the practice you attend if necessary, or consult someone in an alternative field. There is a booklet listing alternatives, many of which are staffed by medically qualified people, if that is what you prefer (see Useful Addresses).

Second, come off gradually, a little at a time. Read one of the guides to withdrawal, such as Shirley Trickett's *Coming off Tranquillizers.*

Do realize that withdrawal symptoms can be very real. They can even seem like those of your original complaint! Here they are: nausea, trembling, panic attacks, pins and needles, 'jelly legs', aches and pains, some severe, feelings of unreality, plus all those mentioned in side effects. They *will* pass.

Do tell close contacts that you're coming off and ask for patience. Take vitamins.

Why have we made such a mess of dealing with stress? Basically because neither contemporary stress-levels nor the means to treat them with tranquillizers have been around for much longer than three or four decades, which is a short time for medical experience. The first real tranquillizer, Largactil, was developed only 30 years ago.

MAKING MORE HEALTH DECISIONS

So we must forgive and forget. But meanwhile we must remove ourselves from the willing 'guinea pig' pen. Taking personal responsibility for our health is the only sensible way to achieve this. Many people felt that tranquillizers were doing them no good long before they thought of discontinuing them. As one patient said 'they just make me worry slower!'

So question your doctor closely if he or she recommends putting you on tranquillizers. There may be a support group you can join instead – or as well – which may help you to minimize the length of time you have to take them.

THE WORST STRESS OF ALL: DEPRESSION AND BEYOND

Depression is an international disease of epic proportions. It is the epidemic of our times, more prevalent than AIDS. Everyone has suffered from it to some degree. What exactly is it?

Depression is stress taken one major stage further. Depression is stress that has gone underground – into the unconscious – to a point at which you no longer have a grip on the whys and wherefores of it, only on the results with which you have been left.

Colour says it all for us. From simply feeling blue or browned off, you suddenly plummet into a world where not only the weather but everything else seems grey. From there it is only one step to black despair, or worse, the blinding white of nothing, like living in snow.

Depression is the illness of our time. Remember, it is just another form of stress, a form that ironically, is more acceptable to live with. Why is this? Because depression is anger turned inwards. When first we are stressed, we get angry at what is stressing us. This is natural. If our car breaks down or public transport is delayed, our first reaction is anger. If you doubt this, recall an occasion when you were going off on holiday and you were told that your flight was delayed. Just when you were about to enjoy yourself, you were thwarted.

Before you accepted the inevitable and talked yourself round, anger was almost undoubtedly your first reaction. You may even remember some energetic and probably younger people on the flight kicking up a fuss. The younger you are, the more this kind of anger shows, which is why young people can be very ugly when thwarted: being in the early stages of the stress of life, they have plenty of energy with which to react. You may also have noted something else: they recovered sooner and started to make their own fun in the airport. The relaxation response is functioning more normally with them, too.

Later, we resign ourselves to things we can't change, either because of experience or simply indifference born of lack of energy. But the sum total of these 'things we can't change' especially if they seem unfair, gets us down. Delayed planes are not the issue now, but unfairness at work, being shabbily treated by a relative or friend, being passed over when we have given our best – that sort of thing.

WHEN DEPRESSION STARTS
The pattern starts in childhood. Unfairness is something that really gets children down. They react angrily, and because anger seems ugly, they are quashed, not listened to. Usually they are reprimanded to boot and told they are to blame. Dejection sets in and they start doubting their

own reactions. This is when anger begins to turn inwards. This is the start of depression.

Of course we cannot always get our own way, we are not always right, and anger is not always justified. But that is the mechanism.

Remember: the negative face of anger is depression. Look back to the beginning of the section on stress, and review the list of triggers that can start a bout of depression. When one of these triggers happens in life, depression can move from being something experienced from time to time, on a few days each month or just after a row, to something that is with you all the time. Like a grey mantle, it covers and colours your every waking moment.

When depression reaches that stage, help is needed. But still people struggle on, because they haven't got any illness as such. This is a mistake. The cure cannot start until you admit that you *are* depressed and need to do something about it. And when you do seek help, don't just rely on your doctor. View that help as getting you over the initial stages of a recovery that is likely to take some time.

Contact a support group. You may think that the last thing you need is to be among more depressed people, but these are the mirrors you need in order to see what you are going through, what you are really like and why your family may be avoiding you or not being sympathetic towards you. You may even start helping those who are depressed and in so doing realize you are not as badly off as some. This has happened before.

Meanwhile, the stages of the cure probably go something like this.

1. A spell on anti-depressants. These are drugs and you need to ask your doctor how and when they should be taken. They are powerful drugs and there are certain things you must not do with them – probably not drink. Since drink is a depressant anyway it would probably be unwise to do so even if you are allowed!

2. A spell off work. This can be a double-edged sword. You may feel you need a rest from all the trials and tribulations, but you also need to have your mind taken off your depression, so struggle in if you can. If you are out of work, struggle to find a little job, different from your regular job if needs be. Even charity work is better than sitting at home and may even lead to a job offer. Don't take turn-downs as personal put-downs. It is a symptom of your illness to do so. If all of these avenues fail, start a creative project at home, make a sweater, build something, however slowly.

3. Try to do one small thing from the list you've got in your head (such as ring a friend, take a coat to the cleaners, have a haircut) every day.

4. Try to get off your pills or reduce them as soon as you can. There

are homoeopathic and herbal remedies that can act as a bridge. (See Useful Addresses for the NMS leaflet.)

BUY one of the following books (or get them from the library) and keep them by you, reading a bit now and then: *Overcoming Depression* by Dr Richard Gillett, *The Joy of Stress* by Dr Peter Hanson and *You Can Heal Your Life* by Louise Hay.

One other important point needs to be made which somehow gets omitted and that is this: when you start getting better you will start to get nasty about little things. This is the anger beginning to come out, and it has to happen. What went in, has to come out. However this can be unpleasant for your friends and family, who are usually convenient butts for it. Here are some alternatives:

1. Take up a sport or exercise, which allows you to express this aggression.
2. Select a chair (possibly belonging to someone in the family who is part of your problem) and kick it hard when they're not around. Take out all your rage on that chair. Thump it with cushions if you don't want the kick-marks to show. Call it by name if you wish (but know that the name is only part-cause of your anger).

Remember: anger is not nice to behold, but it is natural. However, we can't always show it to the prime culprit in our lives – he or she may be contributing to the rent! – but we can let it out from where it lurks in body tissues, hardening walls of arteries, threatening to rupture blood vessels, strip linings from stomachs, twist sexual organs into knots. We may not be able to thump the culprit, but the important thing is to thump something – hard.

There is a very interesting story to be told about this. A counsellor was once given a client who was beating and cutting her children with a kitchen knife. She was informed by the client that she was unable to control bouts of red anger. The counsellor asked if she had a garden. 'A yard, yes' she was told. She suggested that when her client felt these bouts of red anger she should take the knife, go into the yard and stab the ground. The client did so. After a while she stopped stabbing the children. Then she stopped stabbing the ground – she started instead to make holes in it with the knife and to plant things. Her yard became a garden.

This story says much but demonstrates one important truth: anger is not endless. It builds up a head of steam, which has to come out. However if it comes out in a forceful or destructive way it may get blocked before it's out by those witnessing the consequences of it. Then it becomes dammed up again. So stab the ground. It's better than stabbing yourself in the heart, or worse, your nearest and dearest.

DEPRESSION AND THE FAMILY

When depression hits someone, the entire family group is affected by it. What is less accepted is that the whole family group may be responsible for the symptoms, as may well be its family predecessors (parents etc.).

Sometimes the only way to tackle this complex kind of problem with any hope of permanence is to have a family review, under the auspices of a group counsellor. The essential viewpoint that only an outsider can provide is supplied by the counsellor. Guidelines for this and other treatment alternatives are given in the books mentioned above. Information is often available from Citizen's Advice Bureaux.

NERVOUS BREAKDOWN

Generally, stress and depression get better on their own, but occasionally they develop into serious mental breakdown. It is not the purpose of this book to tackle serious illness, other than from the preventive viewpoint. Thus, if stress and depression are recognized and addressed, it is unlikely that anything further will happen.

For those who do go over the edge into nervous breakdown (or fear they are) there is only one thing to say: get help. Do not feel guilty: there is no longer any stigma attached to nervous illness – it is universal. Don't just go to your doctor; contact an organized group of sufferers – they have been there; they can help you find the road to recovery.

EATING DISORDERS AND S.A.D.

It is important to recognize that anorexia and bulimia as well as other eating and some seasonal disorders such as SAD (Seasonal Affective Disorder, see Chapter 9) all have their origins in stress, some going back to childhood. This is all the more reason to recognize stress in the young, and find its causes before they lead to destructive or self-destructive behaviour in adolescence.

STRESS AND CHILDREN

Children suffer from stress every bit as much as adults. Look back at the list of stress symptoms earlier in this chapter, which included trembling, sweating, nervous coughs, fidgeting and upset stomachs, and you will almost invariably be able to recall children close to you suffering from them.

The problem is that stress and the need to relieve it go hand in hand. And with children there is the danger of their relieving it with drugs. If the adults can relieve it by taking tranquillizers, then what's the difference between that and something which has the same effect but gives you a lift too?

Here are some alarming statistics: 30 per cent of 15-year-old children smoke regularly; 250,000 people use heroin in Britain alone – and the figure increases by 30 per cent, nearly one-third, each year; solvent abuse deaths, most involving young children, are rising even more quickly – by nearly 100 per cent in the 1980s.

Authorities who study these matters think that children often learn the drug habit at home. They see domestically used drugs, such as nicotine, tranquillizers and alcohol, and see they are being used to relieve stress. Sometimes they are even given them to keep them quiet. Guilty?

CHILDREN, DIET AND STRESS
There are other alarming factors contributing to stress in children and these are far more insidious.

Number one on the hit-list is the junk diet that most children now insist on eating, thanks to TV advertisements and busy mothers finding such foods quick to prepare. Not only is this empty food, with little or no nutritional value, but it is also dangerously empty because chemicals, sometimes hundreds of them, are being used to give colour, fizz, taste, a boost to the system, instant energy and so on. Many of these chemicals are insidiously poisoning children. There is now a proven link between hyperactivity and highly coloured foods. There are other proven links between behaviour and certain additives in food.

There are now several attested studies of youths in detention centres whose behaviour was completely transformed by a change in diet to healthy, living wholesome foods such as meat and vegetables, salads, food which had been grilled and steamed rather than fried, with little sugar, no fizzy drinks, no hamburgers or French fries.

The people who conducted these studies tried other measures besides diet to see if they had a comparable effect on violent and anti-social behaviour. In one of two detention centres, youths were given a lot of kindness and attention but no change in diet, while in the other the diet was changed to wholesome foods but no extra efforts were made with kindness or attention. The detention centre with the dietary change showed the greater remission of violent and anti-social behaviour.

It is not sufficient to give children a healthy diet – although this will improve both brain function and behaviour (those wanting to know more should read Gwylim Robert's book *Boost Your Child's Brainpower*); it is also necessary that they should learn why it is important to look after their bodies.

An omnipresent threat to the young comes from drugs and drug pushers, and visionary schemes such as the Life Education Programmes (mobile units visit schools to teach young children, in an entertaining way, how to treat their bodies well and why) have been shown to be particularly effective in reducing levels of violent behaviour and drug-taking among adolescents who underwent the training a decade earlier. Life Education Programmes are now available to British schools, as well as to those in their country of origin, Australia (see Useful Addresses).

AND FINALLY TO SLEEP!

Getting a good night's sleep is of such vital importance to people that 5 million tranquillizers and sleeping pills are taken nightly in Britain. No doubt several hundreds of thousands of bottles of alcohol are drained for the same purpose.

Why is sleep evading us? It would seem that our lifestyles no longer contain sufficient physical exercise to tire us out as they did our grandparents. On the other hand, those self-same lifestyles have increased the amount of stressful worries we have.

Do we really need our sleep? The answer to that is most definitely yes, and for two reasons. First, the physical reason: at night during sleep the immune system is extremely active repairing the body cells. However, other systems of the body also have a much needed rest. Heartbeat and respiration slow down, for example, and urine production drops.

Second, the psychological/mental benefits: while we sleep the brain seems to re-charge itself. Interspersed between periods of deep (orthodox) sleep, which appear to be connected with recuperating body tissues, come briefer periods of paradoxical or REM (Rapid Eye Movement) sleep, which seem to be connected with preserving mental stability. These periods are usually associated with dreams, and in some important way dreams help us to resolve our conflicts as well as re-enact and highlight what we are experiencing in life. People deprived of REM sleep quickly lose touch with reality.

REMEDIES FOR SLEEPLESSNESS
Pain is one of the chief causes of sleeplessness, so obviously it is important to seek treatment for any condition that is causing pain.

Alternatives to sleeping pills must be found because they are addictive and because they alter sleep patterns and affect body maintenance.

Because of this it is important to come off sleeping pills gradually so that the body can adjust back to its normal sleep cycles. So cut your pill in half or tip out the powder in your sleeping capsule, reducing it first by a quarter, then by half, and so on. Accept that at first you will not sleep so soundly.

There are a number of herbal sleep inducers which you can ultimately use as a stand-by, such as *valerian*. A teaspoonful infused in a cup of boiling water and taken before bedtime should have you rivalling Rip Van Winkle. Health food shops also stock a variety of gentle herbal sleep inducers.

To actually get to sleep, try the following sequence:

1. Eat some carbohydrate about an hour or two before retiring. This actually triggers the chemical reactions associated with falling asleep.
2. Have a warm (not hot) bath and then get straight into bed. A warm body is a relaxed body.
3. Make sure your bed is comfortable – not too firm, not too soft and with light bedclothes. Then employ one of these techniques:

● Count backwards from 100

● Read a book to make your eyes tired

● Think of all the Christian names you know beginning with a certain letter of the alphabet (don't always start with A!)

The above techniques are ways to trick you into stopping thinking about something which may keep you awake.

Finally, if you can't sleep, don't worry about it. This is more damaging than losing sleep. The self-correcting system will catch up. You may not get as much sleep but it will be deeper.

Here are seven golden rules for getting you into seventh heaven every night.

1. Try to get up and go to bed at the same time each day.
2. Regular early rising gives you a better chance of being tired at the end of the day.
3. Take regular exercise (preferably walking) at least three times a week – every day if possible.
4. Give up smoking and drinking stimulants such as tea, coffee or cola drinks. Certainly don't take these substances at night! And don't eat spicy or indigestible food at that time.
5. Don't watch violent programmes or anything else likely to upset you on television. Don't take or make phone calls that might do likewise. (Tell the caller, or have someone tell them, that you'll phone them back in the morning. Be firm and they'll learn.)

6. Don't be tempted to use alcohol as a sleep inducer, except in extremely moderate amounts; it may get you off to sleep, but it will disturb your sleep rhythm later.

7. Accept yourself as you are: there's nothing you can do about it late at night, anyway!

CHILDREN AND SLEEPLESSNESS

Children suffer from nameless fears of the night, although they can also play on this. But one thing is certain, if they cannot sleep it is no good scolding them or slamming the door on them, as this will only arouse them. So always try to soothe, and if they are small, preferably stay with them until they fall asleep. Leave a night light on as some children are afraid of the dark.

Above all, try to avoid their picking up any concern you may feel about their not sleeping. This may lead to a pattern of worrying about not sleeping which is all too common in adults, and quite destructive of the very activity it seeks to promote!

8
*
THE SKELETAL AND MUSCULAR SYSTEMS

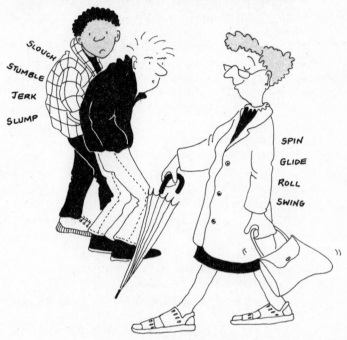

SLOUGH
STUMBLE
JERK
SLUMP

SPIN
GLIDE
ROLL
SWING

YOU ARE AS OLD AS YOUR SPINE......

IN THIS CHAPTER

* Bare facts about bones * Vital role of calcium * Muscles, joints and tendons * Spines and discs * Caring for infant spines * Understanding back pain * Surmounting occupational hazards * Energy and movement * Treatment options (more than you think) * Guidance on back exercises * Sorting out joint problems * Arthritis and gout: dietary solutions * Golden rules of joint care * Controlling osteoporosis * Teeth conservation plan

The saying goes: 'you are as old as your spine'. It is poignantly true. Our image of youth is of uprightness. Our image of old age is of a bent figure. Seldom do we see an upright person who is old, but when we do we sense quite rightly that they are sprightly, alert, and 'young for their age'.

When the spine bends and bows out of shape, the energy flow to the organs and out to the limbs is reduced accordingly. We start to ache and to hold ourselves tense, which further reduces both the blood flow and the vital nerve impulses.

It happens, or so statistics indicate, to nearly all of us. Some 95 per cent of people will get back pain at some time during their lives due to one or other of the bones of the spine.

BONES

As many as 60 million working days each year are lost in the UK on account of those bones in the spine, together with quite a few more on account of joint problems, which render an estimated 1 million people in the United States unemployable at any given time. The picture is no different as far north as Russia or as far south as Australia.

Yet bone is one of the most resilient of the fabrics of life. The tensile strength in compact bones is 700–1,400kg per square centimetre (10,000–20,000lb per sq in) – the same as aluminium or mild steel but lighter and more elastic. Bones are four times stronger than reinforced concrete.

So what goes wrong with this wondrously strong material? Not a lot, usually. The problem is with the joints and other links, such as discs, tendons, ligaments and muscles, that render the body flexible by enabling the bones to be moved.

SWINGS, HOISTS AND PULLEYS
Bones themselves do not move, although they are very much alive, with a plentiful blood supply. However, the muscles pulling on them enable movement, and they achieve this in an elaborate series of expressions of movement, which include spin, glide, roll, swing (flexion and extension of the arm is an example of a swinging movement).

Bones are in the body to give support. There are 206 of them in all, of varying shapes and densities, ranging from the smallest, the anvil in the ear, to the largest, the thigh bone or femur. They afford an amazing 1,200 square metres (1,435 sq yards) of anatomic surface, most of which is accounted for by the myriad carunculations within the bone's surfaces.

These are important to the body since they facilitate one of its major maintenance tasks – which is to constantly repair, reabsorb and rebuild its bones to suit our changing needs and ways of life. And quite apart from this, within the ribs, pelvis and sternum lies the active bone marrow, in which millions of red blood cells are made virtually by the minute.

Bones also act as a storehouse for mineral salts, particularly calcium. In fact, bone would not differ from other connective tissue were it not for the crystals of calcium phosphate that strengthen and rigidify its collagen structure.

THE VITAL ROLE OF CALCIUM

The vital calcium metabolic process that takes place within bone tissue, releasing calcium into the body when needed, storing it when these needs have been met, and deploying and demolishing it to rebuild its own tissues (99 per cent of body calcium is in bones), is one of the key processes of life.

Special cells, called osteoblasts, form collagen (the basic connective tissue of body) and combine it with calcium for strength, when building new bone. Other cells, osteoclasts, break down the collagen and release calcium when breaking it down. It would seem that we have within our bones a symphonic army of wise cells constantly working to meet and maintain our changing demands. Who conducts this wonderful orchestra and what keeps in in tune? Who translates our mechanical needs into a score, a blueprint for rebuilding?

When the calcium metabolism goes wrong or there is insufficient calcium in the diet, bone density suffers and bones start to become brittle and to break. This leads to rickets in youth and, after middle age, to osteoporosis, a widespread complaint that incapacitates many older people. The apparently simple answer – to ingest more calcium – rarely solves the problem after middle age and sometimes compounds it (see below).

However, the increasingly widespread nature of the problem and the seriousness of the symptoms when things go wrong reflect just how important is the role played by healthy bone in maintaining the body's mineral integrity and in particular the calcium balance.

This can be better understood when it is seen that calcium levels are extremely important for the maintenance of neuromuscular perform- ance, interneuronal (nerve) transmission and the integrity and permeab- ility of cell membranes. If nothing gets in or out of cells, toxins build up and vital nutrients are excluded. The cell effectively dies from starva- tion and toxification.

Blood coagulation is affected by calcium levels too. The rigid con- stancy with which calcium levels are maintained in the body (bones are aided in this by hormones and the kidneys and intestines) attests to its biological importance.

MUSCLES

The muscles of the body – 620 that we can move of our own accord plus many more involuntary ones in the heart, blood vessels, intestines and so on that we cannot move or control – comprise as much as 40 per cent of total body weight. They are composed of overlapping bundles of fibres and they are activated by nerve impulses arising in the brain. On an order from the brain their fibres contract in one direction and expand in the other, in perfect coordination, to enable us, for example, to bend an arm or lift a leg to climb stairs. A series of elaborate chemical processes as well as electrical nerve impulses permit them to perform tasks as powerful as chewing food or as delicate as threading a needle.

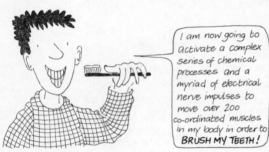

I am now going to activate a complex series of chemical processes and a myriad of electrical nerve impulses to move over 200 co-ordinated muscles in my body in order to BRUSH MY TEETH!

Some muscles are enormously strong: the thigh muscle can produce a tension of 1,180kg (2,600lb)! But strength is not all – coordination is, if anything, more important. No one muscle ever works by itself; it coordinates with other muscles in order to produce the complex set of movements that we take for granted, such as whistling. Some muscles help to keep us erect, while others enable us to bend, twist and turn. The ones that keep us erect are on duty all day, and in the course of a day, we actually shrink, losing a centimetre or two of height due to the pull of gravity and because spinal fluids are forced out from between the vertebrae. When we sleep we replace that vital fluid as well as rest the muscles that keep us upright. For this reason alone, the need for a good night's sleep on a good supportive bed would seem paramount for joint and spinal maintenance.

LIGAMENTS AND CARTILAGE

Bones themselves are bound together by ligaments and their ends are covered with cartilage, which ensures the smooth movement of the 187 joints. There is also a special kind of slippery fluid produced between the joints of bones called synovial fluid, which further facilitates their gliding over each other.

All in all, the bones, ligaments, and muscles comprise the human skeleton as we know it, the flexible scaffold by which we are enabled to stand erect in perfect balance while supporting the tremendous weight of the head – up to 11kg (25lb) – and tissues (weight depending on fatness!).

No wonder such a complex and key structure is prone to the stresses and strains of life's movements, resulting in varying disorders described under such headings as cricks, sprains, strains, twists, breaks, fractures, slips, dislocations, pulls, etc., all of which have one common result, *pain*!

THE SPINE

The linchpin of the skeletal system is, of course, the spine, and its construction is little short of wondrous. Far from being a straight column – such a construction would never be able to bear the weight required of it – the spine actually consists of an S-curve. This doubly bent spring arrangement is far less vulnerable and enables us to pound pavements, sneeze, dance flamenco and perform a variety of other jarring activities without shattering its components.

The lower curve of the spine, a graceful inwards moving one, is called the lumbar lordosis because it involves the lumbar or small of back region. The thorax arches out slightly, and this curve is called the thoracic kyphosis. This is the part of the spine to which the ribs are attached, and it is not surprising to find that this part has the least mobility. Nevertheless, it is sufficiently flexible to allow us to throw a discus or frisby, to pick up a pencil that has fallen down by the side of our chair, or to turn to see what is coming up behind us, while still performing its basic function of assisting the ribs to lift so that we can breathe. The top curve, where the neck arches inwards again, is called the cervical lordosis. If all or any one of these curves gets flattened or distorted there is strain and pain on the structure.

BABY SPINES & THEIR CARE
When a baby is born its spine is relatively straight. The curves slowly develop as it begins to spend more and more time upright. Thus the first year or two are critical for the developing spine, which should never be allowed to bow in an unnatural curve such as happens when baby is wheeled in his or her modern push-chair, stroller or buggy. Old-fashioned prams, which kept baby's spine horizontal, were much healthier. A short trip down to the shops may be fine, but long-term

sojourns in a push-chair, in which baby's back is held in an unnaturally curved position, will not help. As this chapter progresses you will see that our modern lifestyles and habits have much to answer for in respect to increasing spinal problems. Does the term lounge lizard conjure up any spinal pictures?

UNDERSTANDING BACK PAIN

The spine itself consists of 24 tough drum-shaped vertebrae, which facilitate the moving; the other nine are fused, five in the sacral area where the hip bones flare out, and four right down in the base in the tail (actually it is a vestigial tail) called the coccyx. Anyone who has ever fallen on their bottom while learning to roller skate or skidded on the proverbial banana skin to land in a sitting position will know all about the coccyx. Such a fall can often dislodge it from its position and thereby upset the weight distribution of the whole spinal column, since the coccyx is in a balance relationship with the atlas, the top vertebrae of the neck nearest the head: point and counterpoint.

People think that they only hurt one part of the back when they fall or strain it, but in fact referred imbalances can affect the entire spine and its function. That is why referred pain is very common – that is, pain that is not felt in the area where the injury happened but somewhere else.

This is why immobilizing an injured spine can lead to pain and stress elsewhere. The whole edifice needs to move freely for the weight to be borne evenly. This puts a different complexion on wearing a brace or having a disc surgically fused. These last-ditch measures should be considered only when all efforts to rehabilitate the troubled part have failed. Ideally, any therapeutic technique or exercise should encompass the entire spinal column and its mobility – and probably the joints as well.

SPINAL DISCS
Between each vertebra are circular discs or pads of fibrous tissues with a liquid nucleus, constructed rather like a famous brand of chocolate cream mints. These act as the undercarriage, or shock-absorber system, within the spine, and they are extremely strong, despite modern belief to the contrary, as the commonly described complaint 'slipped disc' might suggest. In fact, it is virtually impossible for discs to slip, so strongly are they anchored. However, if unnatural pressure is placed on the discs, caused either by muscles becoming weak and not holding the vertebrae of the spine in place or by strain or injury, cracks may appear in the discs' periphery, and out of these cracks oozes the liquid nucleus matter, to irritate and put pressure on surrounding tissues, just

as cracks in the shell of the above-mentioned chocolate creams would allow the centre filling to ooze out.

However, this rarely happens overnight, as some dramatic stories seem to suggest – 'I was just putting on my tights when. . . '. The final indignity, often slight, is the last of many straws that the back has previously absorbed. Which is why early twinges must always be heeded and an exercise programme to strengthen the spine worked out.

THE SPINAL CORD

The bony spine houses and protects the all-important spinal cord. If, through injury, this cord is broken, paralysis below the point of the break occurs. The spinal cord does not in fact extend all the way down the spine, but stops at the second lumbar vertebra, somewhere near the small of the back. After that point the nerves trail downwards to feed the legs and lower organs.

The spinal cord, of course, has a direct link with the brain, which is housed and protected in another bony protective shell – the cranium. Although this seems like one bone there are in fact 29 bones in the head fitted together like jig-saw pieces, yet they are moveable. In common with all bones a lifetime of sculpturing goes on to accommodate our needs.

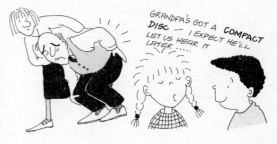

Emerging from the spinal column in pairs between each vertebra are the nerve branches, which feed the entire body. There are 43 pairs of these, 12 cranial and 31 spinal. It is easy to imagine how pressure on any one of them, caused by a minute displacement of a bone in the spine or elsewhere, could result in anything ranging from vague discomfort to severe pain, felt wherever the nerve ends or the nerve begins, so the symptoms, like Shakespeare's description of Cleopatra, are possessed of 'infinite variety'. At best the insidious effect of this on the body will result in degrees of tiredness.

BACKS AGAINST THE WALL OF CONTEMPORARY LIFE

Never before have we demanded so much of our spines for so little. Modern lifestyles are far more sedentary than those of our forebears.

Labour-saving gadgets are exactly as described, they save labour, which means they save movement – all the stretching, bending movements that the spine thrives on. Spines must bend in order to be healthy. Like the hinge on a rarely used door, joints both in the spine and in the limbs become rusty if not used. No wonder that there are more spinal complaints from 25–30 year olds than ever before, according to back experts and therapists. Sedentary lifestyles and fat-producing diets are considered to be two main contributory factors.

Modern sports are not good for the spine either, so back experts say. All too often these consist of a series of repetitive movements that do not fully extend the capacity of the joint because precision and accuracy in the sport require economy and control of the movement. Take ballet, for example. The exquisite control demanded of ballet movements is not good for the back, which needs to work in a much more free and easy way. Many ballet dancers have bad backs. Take tennis. One arm is required to do all the work while holding a heavy racket at the end of its length, while the rest of the body tries desperately to keep up with it. Forehand strokes are more common than backhand, the result being that one muscle group works more than the other – the common result, tennis elbow.

Rugby players end up injured wrecks, too, from all that weight, all those collisions, and all that flying and falling. And now that there have been three decades of joggers, American research has shown that the constant pounding does terrible things to the spine and joints. We really have to rethink our entire exercise regime if we want to spend the last few decades of our lives in anything but pain. And what a pity. That's just when we've got the money and freedom to enjoy ourselves.

Below is a list of sports considered good and bad by modern back experts such as Sarah Keay, the author of a 'must' for back sufferers, *Back in Action*.

Bad: tennis, rugby, squash, golf, jogging – in fact any sport that demands much of a few muscles and too little of others plus any sport that requires sudden or repetitive movements that could sprain and strain the body.
Good: yoga (top seal of approval since it stretches and strengthens all muscles), table tennis (the bat is small and light, the movements many and varied), aerobics programmes (but only with careful progress).
Middle-of-the-road: swimming, soccer.
Note: do not equate the undoubted benefits of exercise that makes the heart beat faster with exercise that strengthens and stretches the spine. Any exercise is good for the circulatory system, providing it is done on a regular basis. The spine is more demanding of its exercise programme.

HOW BACK PAIN BEGINS

A well-known osteopath (more about osteopathy later) once told me his principle of treatment: 'find it, fix it, forget about it.' Like all wise sayings this one has its limitations and qualifications, of which I am sure the osteopath in question was aware.

A typical scenario of how back pain starts goes something like this. When we move, an elaborate series of muscle movements orchestrates our desired move – some extending, some flexing, some rotating and some twisting – all of which work perfectly until or unless we catch the muscles unawares by a snatched movement or an unexpected jar, such as stepping off a pavement which is higher than we thought, or being jolted in public transport.

The result is a shock wave that passes through the joints in question. If these happen to be the vertebrae, most of the time other vertebrae help them to ride it out, but sometimes this is not the case, and a rick or strain occurs.

Whenever a joint gets strained it weeps. Fluid (blood and lymph) oozes out as if an internal cut had occurred. These fluids do, in fact, bring to the site essential materials for the healing process, but they also cause swelling, and the swelling in turn presses on nerves and causes pain.

As a result, we sense the soreness and hold ourselves taut in that area. A whole pattern of muscle spasm is set up in order to protect the area from further movement. This is fine, but regrettably the spine stores the incident, as do the muscles. Muscles have memories. Any future movement they perform in that area will be affected by the incident. In time this may well pass, although the strained joint may retain some stiffness because the muscles continue to protect its movement past the crisis stage.

If at some future date this weak link is further aggravated, an ever-worsening pattern of stiffness and soreness will take place, with life-giving blood unable to penetrate the stiffened tissues to deliver oxygen and nutrients and take debris away.

Unfortunately, tissue starved of blood starts to degenerate and this is when discs can become starved of nutrients and begin to lose their elasticity and bounce. Death in the body doesn't just happen when we die. It can occur in bits and pieces all over the place. Our constant vigilance is needed. For that reason and that reason alone, never protractedly nurse or ignore an injury.

Fear, of course, can make the above scenario worse because fear stiffens muscles, too. Cold can do likewise, which is why we always try to keep an injury warm.

Regrettably, such progressive weakening can eventually extend to other vertebrae until a really serious situation occurs. One or two discs may become impacted or completely degenerated, and at that stage the person is usually in a great deal of pain – not exactly from the discs, because discs have very few nerves, but because the shrunken disc has allowed too much play in the surrounding vertebrae, which then tend to move out of line. The classic description of this is 'I've put my back out'.

PAIN: CHIEF DIAGNOSTIC TOOL

Back pain is hard to diagnose, as every back expert knows. This is partly because of the phenomenon mentioned above, referred pain – i.e. pain felt in another area from the actual cause of the problem – and partly because of the variety of pain that back problems can initiate, from the stabbing shooting pain of sciatica, to the dull diffuse pain of dural trouble (the dura is the protective lining of the spinal cord itself).

Until the source of the pain is found, simply treating the pain is not addressing the cause, merely alleviating that most valuable of all signs, the symptom. In fact, to relieve back symptoms it is often as effective to take a muscle relaxant as a pain-killer or anti-inflammatory drug, because the tensed bunch of muscles around the problem area is likely to be compounding the felony. However, relaxants are no more treating causes than pain killers. Both should be used for short-term alleviation only – eliminating such medications puts an added burden on elimination systems of the body such as the kidneys, which could, in fact, make back pain worse. It is well known to back experts that lumbago, back pain in the lumbar region, is often made worse by kidneys not functioning optimally.

SEEKING TREATMENT: THE VARIOUS OPTIONS

The poor beleaguered patient usually goes first to the doctor, who tells them to rest (see below), gives them anti-inflammatories, muscle relaxants or pain-killers and may or may not investigate further by taking X-rays, depending on his or her assessment of the gravity of the pain.

Unfortunately X-rays don't show movement restriction, any more than a picture of a hinge shows how it is working. Sometimes it looks the worst where it doesn't hurt!

OSTEOPATHY AND CHIROPRACTIC

Others suffering pain go immediately to an osteopath or chiropractor to be manipulated. Actually, unless care is exercised, they may be doing themselves more harm than good. If it is a new back problem, caused by a known recent event (the more recent the better), then the chances are that the therapist will be able to find it, fix it and then you will be able to forget it. With luck your therapist will forget it too and not keep you going back for more and more manipulations, thereby weakening the entire spinal structure and setting you up for even more manipulations.

What you really want is to get to someone who will not do anything drastic until you and they are confident that they have found the site of your pain and have a pretty good idea about its cause. Most good back people say they just have to put their hands on a back to know where the problem lies. The secret is to find out a good back person before you need them.

Only a minority of back problems is best addressed by chiropractic or traditional osteopathy in which manipulation is always done, because the problem with manipulation is that the conditions under which it is done have to be timed to the second, with the patient ready and the manipulator ready. The degree of strength needed must be judged exactly – a frail female and a hefty male will need vastly different degrees of this, and this highly complex set of conditions cannot be met every time.

That said, there are times when manipulation is called for, and the motto should be, with a sudden injury, the sooner the better. Everyone has heard of stories of people being carried into osteopaths doubled up and walking out cured. We hear less of the stories where people have been made worse, mainly by overtreatment and too harsh a technique.

Resting an injury is now a dirty word among most knowledgable back experts. Apart from the initial 24 or 48 hours, to allow the initial swelling and soreness to abate, rest simply encourages the joint to stiffen and collect deposits. For this reason doctors now insist that physiotherapy begins very shortly after a broken limb is set. Obviously with a bad injury expert advice must be sought and taken, but it is as well to know that there are two distinct schools of thought regarding backs and joint injuries and the modern school says gently bend it. Keep it moving. *Use it or lose it*.

MANUAL MOBILIZATION
Manual mobilization is one of the newest approaches to backs. It speaks for itself. Recognizing the value of hands-on touch for health beliefs, the therapist gently (and sometimes not so gently) kneads the spine in order to get the entire framework mobile. Manipulation involving cracking is considered unnecessary in most cases. If muscles are relaxed and tissues gently stretched, joints will find their own way back into place. Most experts trained in this method come from the school of physiotherapists, though not all. Central registers of physiotherapists may carry names of those trained in this way.

CRANIAL OSTEOPATHY

Cranial osteopathy (strictly speaking sacro-cranial osteopathy) follows a divergent pathway from techniques described above since it arises from a different principle – that is, that information can be brought to bear about the condition of the spine by feeling the sacro-cranial rhythm.

This is one of the basic rhythms of life originating in the brain. It is more basic than breathing, and its minute pulsation is conveyed throughout the brain and spinal cord by delicate fluctuations in the cerebro-spinal fluid. The cranial osteopath tunes into this for special information about the state of play in the skeletal system anywhere in the body. Treatment is extremely gentle; while most forms of osteopathy and chiropractic end at the neck, it incorporates delicate movements of the bones of the cranium, since arguably those bones can be displaced just like any others. In fact, cranial osteopaths believe that a wide range of symptoms such as persistent head pain, congestion, dental and bite problems, a nose or eye which runs on one side but not the other, as well as many problems to do with the senses (tinnitus, problems with smell, etc.) may be alleviated by gentle manipulation of the head bones. Arguably, they say, the very nature of our lives sets us up for some kind of fall or blow to the head, during which any one of the 29 bones can be infinitesimally misplaced. Major blood vessels course through the head, supplying vital nutrients and oxygen. These can be compromised, as can nerves.

Much of the cranial osteopath's work is done on the newly born who have suffered long and difficult deliveries, especially with forceps. Many a baby suffers from pain from this largely unrecognized source, and many a face is distorted for life during those vital first moments of existence.

Cranial osteopaths are always represented within a group or association (see Useful Addresses). Qualifications and training should be considered when making your choice, but as with all forms of osteopathy, it is as well to use the senses when choosing them too. Like all musicians, these musicians of the spine are born, not made.

ACUPUNCTURE

This technique works extremely well for all types of back problems, even those which osteopathy cannot treat, such as arthritic and diseased spines. Acupuncture tunes up and opens the energy channels of the body which often become blocked during the course of spinal debilitation. However, it does not interfere with the structure and therefore cannot exacerbate disease. Often the gentle stimulation it gives is enough to trigger the body's natural defences to take up the fight against whatever spinal problem exists. Once again, registered associations will provide names of practitioners in your area, and once again you are advised to sift carefully. It seems to be a feature of people with bad backs that they become so desperate they will try almost anyone or anything to get relief. Many bad backs are overtreated as a result of this.

THE ALEXANDER TECHNIQUE

This therapy sometimes works very well with backs, especially if the problem is one of posture or the way in which some movement is made. In fact, it is a re-education in movement, based on the fact that we often use our bodies badly, and this leads to distortions which can cause injury.

At the end of normally 30 lessons, you are much more aware of the balance of your head, neck and spine. You will have been shown how to do the simplest things: sitting in a chair, walking across a room. We spend so long in distorted postures that it is hard work at first educating the muscles, but after that moving without tension and strain become second nature (see Useful Addresses).

EXERCISES

Anyone wanting to learn about back exercises should read Sarah Keay's book mentioned above. She recommends a back block to help loosen up the spinal joints, and the address for this simple piece of equipment is in her book. However, an even simpler tennis ball (a new one) will

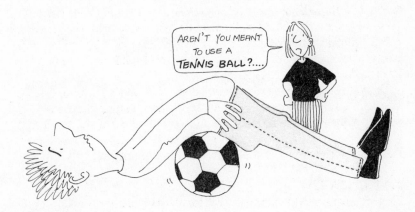

suffice. Just lower your back gently onto it and roll it round the stiff bit. There are also an excellent series of illustrated exercises in Jan de Vries' book *Neck and Back Problems*. With all these techniques start slowly and cautiously – Rome was not built in a day.

STRENGTHENING THE STOMACH MUSCLES

Many experts agree that problems and pain in the back (especially the lower back) often come from poorly toned stomach muscles. It is the stomach muscles that hold the back in place. 'Sit-ups' are traditionally the way to strengthen stomach muscles but back sufferers must beware. Begin slowly. Do not attempt to actually sit up – just raising your shoulders from the floor lying on your back, (arms crossed over chest) can begin to strengthen the stomach muscles. If you are undergoing back treatment or therapy, check with your therapist before starting any exercise programme. Ideally, it is better to be shown how to do exercises than to pick them up in books.

Here are some more tips for people with 'backs'.

● Never sit in a straight-backed chair (you need a slight bow) nor in a deep, spongy chair or sofa without plenty of cushions to support the small of your back.

● Choose a firm mattress, not one that allows you to sink into it. Or put a board under your present mattress.

● Pick up and carry objects by holding them close to your chest. Bring the waiting chest down to the object, not the object up to the chest! Don't snatch the weight, don't twist the spine, and take it slowly.

● Try not to bend forwards when working or walking.

● On waking, get down on hands and knees and do a cat arch and careful dip.

● Never sit or stand for a long time without getting up and walking around for a bit.

● Keep your back warm.

● Never despair. Keep moving, you are pumping blood into your joints. Don't fear pain: pain won't incapacitate you but inactivity might – and lead to more pain.

JOINTS AND JOINT PROBLEMS

A joint is a structure that separates two or more adjacent elements of the skeleton. The heads of joints close together are covered with a slippery substance, cartilage, which enables them to glide over each other without friction. This movement is further facilitated by the egg-white-like synovial fluid.

Joints are held together by *ligaments*, which are tough elastic fibres of collagen. It is actually these which enable the joint to bend. Between two joints that glide over each other are *bursas*, sacs containing synovial fluid which further cushion joint movement and absorb the stresses. They are also found where *tendons* pass by bony areas (tendons are rigid and do not stretch like *cartilage* because their purpose is to hold bony structures in place).

All these terms will be familiar to anyone who has had joint injuries, some of the most common of which are housemaid's knee, tennis or golf elbow, frozen shoulder and soldier's heel. As these terms suggest, they are encountered where there is excessive and continual demand on a joint for a specific type of activity. At some stage or other the joint gets pulled by a sudden or excessive movement or strained by not being able to work in all of its directions, or simply over-used. Sometimes this is called by the well-known term *bursitis*, that is, inflammation of the sac protecting the joint.

It is interesting to conjecture that there may be psychological as well as mechanical causes to such joint afflictions. Anything occupational is bound at times to induce stress, and many of these movements are caused by the occupational necessity of frequent use, some of it no doubt resented (soldier's heel?) or performed under the tension of wanting to do well (golfer's elbow?).

Some psychologists suggest to us that frozen shoulder (which ironically affects twice as many women as men – perhaps because they suppress agression more) has in its origins, which may date back as far as childhood, a desire to hit out or protect oneself, its onset in adulthood (often sudden) being precipitated by an event which stirs up the original emotions. 'Shouldering burdens' is another avenue to explore.

The medical profession is considering 'constitutional predispositions' as one cause for such afflictions, since one's constitution is inevitably bound up with one's personality and emotions. It is an interesting avenue to investigate, one which could be pursued by anyone suffering chronically from such an effect. When, under therapy, the emotion is found, tracked down and re-enacted, it can release the expressive muscular pattern which has become quite literally 'frozen' into the joint.

Most joint experts now agree that the important thing about joints is to work them in every way, not just the grooved way demanded by the lifestyle chosen. It is equally important not to neglect an injury. If one group of muscles is used far more than others, exercise of some activity should be chosen (such as yoga) which will disperse the intensity of this by extending other muscles.

JOINT DISEASE AND HOW TO CONTROL IT

Diseases of the joints are more serious, and although rarely life-threatening, probably cause more invalidism in Western countries than any other condition except probably heart disease. Surveys in the UK and USA indicate that as much as 40–50 per cent of the adult population have X-ray-visible signs of arthritis in the joints of the hands and feet. This represents MILLIONS of people, and the degree of affliction increases with age. It is estimated that 175,000 Americans require assistance for even their elementary hygiene because of degenerative hip disease.

Contributory causes are listed as recurrent small athletic or occupational injuries, lifting heavy weights (including the omnipresent one – obesity) and dietary and endocrine factors, which are themselves no doubt largely dependent on dietary factors.

It is the dietary factors to which we can turn with the greatest hope of salvaging this situation. But first a brief look at arthritis, and what it is in its varying forms.

Arthritis is inflammation of the joints of the body, caused either by wear and tear or by disease. It is a general term that covers many different complaints of the joints and it is very important for sufferers to know what kind of arthritis they have, since successful treatment, especially alternative forms of treatment, will depend upon it.

Rheumatoid arthritis is chronic inflammation of the joints, usually beginning with the smaller joints of the body, and usually beginning before 40 years of age. Approximately 80 per cent of sufferers are women. In addition to the joint symptoms there is usually inflammation of small blood vessels, and the sufferer may have symptoms connected with inflammation of certain body membranes such as the pericardium (enclosing the heart) and the pleura (covering the lungs). It is now being thought of as an auto-immune disease – that is, a disease in which the function of the body's immune system becomes distorted and turns on itself.

Other, less common forms of arthritis closely associated with this disease-profile are psoriatic arthritis and lupus.

Osteo-arthritis is a non-inflammatory disease of the joints, and it usually affects the larger, weight-bearing joints, such as the hip. It is a disease of wear and tear, which affects older people, although it should be said that it is probably present in most but the very young.

Arthritis of the spine is called *spondylitis*. Regardless of the cause or type of arthritis, the process is similar. First there is inflammation, causing pain, stiffness and swelling, then fluid accumulates in the joint. Such chronic inflammation progressively destroys first joint cartilage, then underlying bone, causing adhesions and deformities, which render movement increasingly difficult.

Other types of arthritis include *gout*, which is caused by a build up of tiny crystals of uric acid in the joints that are in turn attacked by the body's immune system. The cells cannot absorb the crystals and die, releasing necrotic fluids into the joints, which inflame them. Gout sufferers are usually fond of foods which contain a lot of purine, such as meat, fish, peanuts, chocolates, alcohol, sugar and salt – in other words a rich diet. These prove too much for the body to cope with from time to time (a stressful event often triggers a gout attack), and the build-up of uric acid which results in its being crystallized out of the blood begins the process.

There is so clearly a diet-related connection with gout that it is one of the easiest forms to control – except in rare circumstances when gout is actually a symptom of another, underlying disease. The solution is to stay off rich food.

All types of arthritis can be helped by diet and the following programme of care.

● Try to avoid, and never ignore, small athletic and occupational injuries.

● Do not lift heavy weights unless you are protected by a pelvic belt or fully aware of what you are doing and how to do it with least strain. So many of us snatch at a weight which has to be lifted, in a kind of martyred rage. Plan ahead – use a wheelbarrow, a trolley, baby's push-chair. Always carry the weight close to the chest, not out in front or dangling from one arm. Bend the knees, not the back, when lifting.

● Obesity. If you have arthritis or a tendency to rheumatism (rheumatism by the way, is simply painful joints, tendons, ligaments and so on, which comes and goes, rather than progresses), consider how important it is to take the load off your joints. However, since there is nearly always emotional involvement in arthritis (daily frustration, worry, fear, long-term unhappy or unfulfilled relationship), it is better to go on eating than to add another misery to your long list of miseries! However, you can at least eat the right things and not the wrong ones. Put in a nutshell: avoid tinned, packeted, processed, dyed, artificially-coloured and flavoured foods. Very little citrus fruit. Never rhubarb. Water should be bottled or purified.

RAW FOOD AND ARTHRITIS
The Royal Free Hospital in London carried out a widely publicized experiment on diet and arthritis. It proved beyond any doubt that a diet high in raw foods greatly alleviated the symptoms of arthritis. The diet should consist of more salads and vegetables than fruit. Raw grated cabbage, grated carrot and raw vegetable juices (freshly extracted) can

go a very long way to helping arthritics. Ideally, 75 per cent of their food should be eaten raw. Regrettably, most arthritics like the very foods that are bad for them – acid-forming foods such as pork, beef and processed meats, shellfish, white bread, jams, cakes, sweets, pastries, buns, pasta, pickles, cheese, chocolate, eggs, coffee, red wine, vinegar and things preserved in it, sugar and salt. All these foods should be avoided.

There are substitutes for most of the foods listed above. A wonderful variety of herb teas and beverages can replace strong tea and coffee; jacket potatoes can replace chips; brown rice can replace polished rice; stoneground wholemeal bread or rye crispbread can replace white bread; honey, molasses or brown sugar can replace white sugar, although never in large quantities. Salads can be dressed with cold-pressed olive or avocado oil, lemon juice or cider vinegar (not salad dressings or mayonnaise); salt substitutes can mostly replace table salt; a few dates or raisins or hunza apricots (dried whole with the stone) can be eaten when something sweet is craved; muesli can replace cornflakes or other cereals; olive oil or a cold-pressed oil, such as sunflower or soya, can replace fat, butter or margarine for cooking.

Think of vegetables, the fresher the better, as your friends, and have a vegetable soup on the go all the time, containing grated carrots, onions, garlic, celery, spinach, turnips and so on. Crudités can help stave off the desire for biscuits and sweet snacks, salads can be a varied and attractive alternative to stodge for lunch. Low-fat cottage cheese can replace richer cheeses in the diet for cheese-lovers.

Your local health store will stock many attractive foodstuffs which are safe for you to eat. Dietary advisors are usually in on a Saturday and the service is free.

NATURAL REMEDIES FOR ARTHRITIS

Evening primrose oil (up to three 500mg tablets a day) has proved helpful for arthritics, who should try to take a 'marine' oil supplement on a daily basis as well (cod liver, halibut or EPA) in addition to basic vitamins and minerals (see Chapter 4). Echinaforce and Symphosan (see Useful Addresses) help some arthritics. Other natural remedies worth trying are green-lipped mussel extract, or a remedy called Cho Jukai (shark liver oil) on which some impressive studies have been carried out. Do give each one a chance – one month's supply is not enough; you should try them for 3 months.

A simple remedy for reducing the acidity from which all arthritics suffer is to juice a raw potato first thing every morning and drink this juice. Grating the potato and squeezing the juice out is second best, but really every arthritis sufferer should invest in a good juicer (Useful

Addresses). Carrot and celery juice (add one green apple to improve the flavour if you wish) should be taken daily. Do not juice ahead and save – juice must be drunk within 20 minutes of preparation in order to get full benefit from its live goodness.

ARTHRITIS AND THE ENVIRONMENT

Examine all environmental factors around you. Are you walking around in rubber shoes on concrete covered floors? You may be cutting off the earth's rays without which we would all sicken and die. Sleep lying north/south; this direction is more in tune with the Earth's energy flow and may render it more accessible to you.

Are you living close to a motorway or high-tension power line? Are you spending too much time too close to the television, or working too long with a word processor?

Are you in a damp climate? Try to wear warm clothing and keep the air inside your dwelling warm. Try wearing a copper bracelet.

All environmental factors must be investigated and minimized where arthritis has developed.

DRUGS AND ARTHRITIS

Regrettably, the drugs prescribed for arthritis have deleterious effects on the immune system, particularly the body's enzyme production. Cortisone, for example, although giving immediate relief, actually throws the body into a constant state of stress, in which calcium may be moved around to be lodged in the wrong parts of the body. In addition, the body's natural production of cortisone dries up. So it is much better to encourage the body to do its own job by giving it the necessary raw materials.

Note: do not immediately stop taking your drugs; in time you may be able to wean yourself gently from them, a fraction at a time. In the meantime there are many things you can take that will to some extent replace what the effect of the drugs is supressing.

Enzyme treatment is one of these. All too often the drugs given suppress the body's production of enzymes. These active substances bring about all the reactions on which life depends, but drugs such as tranquillizers and antihistamines can suppress this activity. Aspirin and anti-inflammatory drugs cause their own set of problems – gastric upsets and dizziness, for example.

For enzyme therapy you will need to go to a naturopath or someone who specializes in the dietary aspects of alternative medicine. You will not be given more drugs. You will be given things that help your body to function at a fundamental level. Previously, treatment for arthritis, like so much orthodox treatment, has been directed towards the management of the symptoms. The actual disease, or its cause, has lain unaddressed. Now there is a glimmering of understanding of how the causal factors may be rectified, and this lies in slowly correcting the faulty body metabolism that has brought about the disease. *

ENERGY, MOVEMENT AND ARTHRITIS

In addition to dietary factors, there are several forms of treatment that help the arthritic person to keep moving and to improve the flow of life-bringing energy.

Biomagnetic therapies are proving particularly effective. All life is vibration (see Chapter 12). Every cell in our bodies is vibrating to a particular tone or key. If that vibration gets off-key through distortion of the body metabolism, disease can result. Vibrational therapies such as tens, diapulse, ultrasound (often used in joint injuries and bursitis) and soft laser are based on re-instating and re-tuning the body's basic vibrations. Electro-crystal therapy is one of the newer vibrational therapies and is usually effective with joint problems (see Useful Addresses). Copper and zinc bracelets also work on the principle of vibratory rectification.

Acupuncture can also open the channels and help clear the body's energy circuits, after which they sometimes correct themselves, but in cases where disease has incapacitated the body, it may have to be prompted to 'remember'. There is nothing dangerous or harmful about such treatments – unlike X-rays they will never do harm, and they may do a great deal of good.

With arthritis it is a question of trying everything to see which link is your particular missing link. Miraculous alleviation is sometimes seen when this missing link is found and provided.

One other very fine therapy which can be done by a family member at home is reflexology. This is gentle all-over foot massage, missing no area of the foot, never being rough, but particularly prodding and kneading any sore spots that are found.

An expert will, of course, achieve far better results and more quickly than an untrained person, but basically this is a treatment that can alleviate pain and cause no harm. Energy zones in the body surface at the feet, and treating the feet is tantamount to treating internal organs, dispersing inflammation and encouraging the flow of vital energy to the tissues. Energy zones surface in the hands as well and gently kneading one's own hands and fingers can help.

The basic rule in arthritis is to keep going. Keep up with the modern literature, often found in a good health magazine (which will also supply you with the addresses of qualified therapists for treatments such as those described above).

RELIEVING THE PAIN OF ARTHRITIS

Some arthritics find that taking a course of epsom salts baths helps their pain. Empty a 1.8kg (4lb) box into one quarter of a tub of hot water.

After 15 minutes immersed in water as hot as you can take it, slowly mix in cool water and stay in the bath of cool water for a few minutes. Dry yourself briskly. Sip a glass of warm water with the juice of a lemon in it and get into bed. This procedures enhances sleep and helps to break down uric acid deposits. Do this nightly for a week, then every other night for a week, then twice weekly. Do not try this treatment if you have cardiovascular disease or high blood pressure. However you can try skin brushing (see Chapter 10).

OSTEOPOROSIS, CALCIUM METABOLISM AND HRT

Osteoporosis, a disease in which calcium is progressively leached out of the bones, which then become porous and brittle, affects an enormous number of people – one in ten men and one in four women. It is by far the most common bone disease, although it is often silent until a brittle bone such as the hip or wrist fractures, often after the slightest injury or fall.

The effects of such fractures are said to incapacitate 22,000 women a year in the UK, 9,000 of whom will die as a result of complications after such fractures. The misery it causes in old people who are thereafter unable to get about is a major contributor to suffering in the old.

In women it is often associated with the menopause since the drop in oestrogen levels that occurs then greatly accelerates the process. Oestrogen prevents the resorption of bone, and its administration after the menopause in the form of hormone replacement therapy (HRT) is of great value in the control of this disease. There are many other advantages in taking HRT as well (see Chapter 9).

Throughout life, bone is built up and reabsorbed by the body according to our required needs. As we become less and less active, the body perceives these needs as lessening. Exercise, especially weight-bearing exercise, is therefore terribly important. A brisk walk of half an hour a day may be all that is needed, but it does help stave off this most unpleasant condition.

Since calcium features very importantly in the build-up and breakdown of bone, it is actually loss of calcium that causes them to become brittle. However, taking a calcium supplement after middle age must be done with care. A very complex set of glandular and hormonal activities needs to be functioning correctly for the calcium to be laid down in bone and not deposited in other less desirable places such as the walls of the arteries. Calcium citrate is the most easily absorbed form of calcium, but it must be taken with magnesium, otherwise soft-tissue calcification, in the walls of the arteries, for example, is likely to occur rather than replacement of bone. Combined with HRT, this policy will help to safeguard against osteoporosis. Vitamin D, which is made by the body in sunlight, is needed too. Regrettably, many older people spend a lot of time indoors and become deficient in this vitamin.

The long-term taking of cortico-steroids also prompts the process of osteoporosis. Many sufferers of arthritis who have been taking steroids find themselves with this added complication. This is all the more reason to try to correct arthritis at ground-roots level with diet and a reduction in acid-forming foods. Fruit (except citrus in this case), vegetables and seeds provide the necessary alkaline climate for bone formation.

TEETH – A VITAL PART OF THE SKELETON

Finally a word about care of the teeth. It is vitally important to floss your teeth regularly and to have plaque removed periodically by a dental hygienist. Keeping bacteria in the mouth down to acceptable levels means less invasion of the body, less gum disease, less misery in latter years trying to eat with fewer (or no) teeth. We would not think of going out in the morning without cleaning ourselves, yet so many of us neglect to clean properly that which should last us a lifetime – our teeth.

Furthermore, mercury (silver fillings) are poisonous – more so for some than others. Some fillings slowly 'leak' small quantities of mercury into the system, and this can undermine the immune function. If you are suffering from any conditions associated with lowered immune function (arthritis is one, candida is another) have your fillings checked either by a kineseologist (see Useful Addresses) or by a dentist using one of the new diagnostic scanners (such as Vega; see Useful Addresses under Centre for Complementary Medicine), which measure the body's delicate electrical energy in relation to foreign substances, foods, medicines and so on. If there is any doubt, it is best to have your silver fillings replaced by inert white fillings. Never allow a dentist to put new 'silver' fillings into your mouth.

Fluoride is also more toxic than is publicly admitted and can cause mottling on teeth of young children. Eliminate this toxin and choose herbal toothpastes. Far too much goes into commercial brands of toothpaste (and into our mouths) about which we know little or nothing. Do you want a three-times-a-day diet of chalk, binders, detergents, lubricants, flavourings and (more than likely) fluoride?

It is the little health measures, those small changes about which we wrote in the introductory chapters, that can make the difference between zip and zap.

9

*

THE ENDOCRINE AND REPRODUCTIVE SYSTEMS

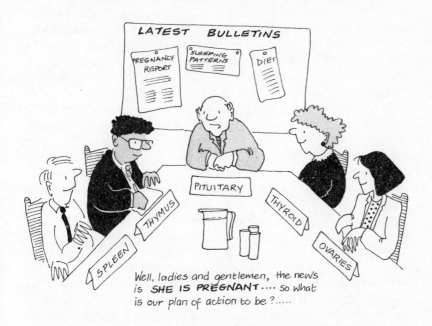

Well, ladies and gentlemen, the news is **SHE IS PREGNANT** ···· so what is our plan of action to be ?·····

IN THIS CHAPTER

✱ The seven glands of vitality ✱ Hormones, your chemical messengers ✱ Adrenal health *v.* salt, pee pills and beta-blockers ✱ Your third eye and SAD ✱ The semi-endocrines ✱ Your sex glands and health ✱ Impotence and infertility ✱ Preventing prostate problems ✱ Making PMT a thing of the past ✱ Preparing for pregnancy ✱ Pros and cons of the Pill ✱ Beating cystitis and thrush ✱ Why VD clinics are VG places ✱ Infertility ✱ Managing the menopause (and other ills) with HRT

The fact that many rejuvenating treatments are directed at the glands of the body indicates just how important they are. Glands secrete substances which aid body functions, such as the sweat glands, which help us to lose heat through evaporation from the skin when we are exercising or in the tropics, or salivary glands, which secrete digestive juices when we eat.

These kinds of glands squirt their substances into the local site of action. But there is another, vitally important group of seven glands called the endocrine glands, whose substances are released directly into the bloodstream, and they can have a widespread effect.

Said to be attached to the seven chakras, or energy-centres of the body, the substances they release are hormones, or chemical messengers, and some 50 of them have been identified in the body, although only a handful of these have key importance in our lives. There is no doubt that their production, which in turn depends on the healthy functioning of the glands that secrete them, is an important determinant of ageing.

The glands of the body, together with the nervous system, control body workings; in fact, a large portion of the endocrine system is under nervous control, and in the case of the endocrine system this is specifically masterminded from an area of the brain called the hypothalamus.

Immediately we begin to suspect a link between thought and glandular activity, and we are right to do so. All glands work on a feedback system, but a modifying influence on such systems is what is being fed into them in the first place!

Most people have heard of the 'fight or flight' syndrome, the body's reaction to stress; most may even have heard that it is to do with adrenaline being released into the system under stressful conditions, such as fright, fear, hurt etc. But not as many may know that this is directly militated through the action of the adrenal glands, which are part of the endocrine system and which are probably the most over-worked glandular reaction in the entire body! (Stress, and what it does to us long-term, is fully explored in Chapter 7.)

GLANDULAR FUNCTIONS AND REPRODUCTION

There is no doubt that one of the prime functions of glands is to help us cope with changes in our environment. But side by side with this, and interacting with it, runs another prime function, and that is to help us maintain our internal environment and its rhythms, in particular reproduction. Often the first sign that our endocrine system is under stress is reflected in problems with the reproductive system (see later). These should never be ignored, however slight they seem – increasingly troublesome PMT, for instance – because they are the body's early warning signs that not enough attention is being paid to the healthy functioning of the glands.

Because their action is so powerful, their malfunction is equally noticeable, and as such they provide vital clues as to where we are on the good health spectrum. Health to illness, like a colour swatch for paints, is a spectrum, ranging from the most vivid (good health) to the palest of shades, representing illness – note how we describe not being well as 'looking pale' or 'white', or 'drained of colour' (see Chapter 12).

TYPES OF HORMONES

Hormones express vital parts of the genetic message and are of various chemical types, many of which are manufactured from that scapegoat of modern health badinage, cholesterol, which is in fact a scapegoat only when overproduced due to excesses in our modern diet, such as too many sweets or fats.

The types may be proteins or peptides, which are formed from amino acids, the building blocks of the body, or glycoproteins, which consist of two key dietary ingredients, proteins and carbohydrates, or aromatic compounds, or the very well-publicized steroids often given to athletes and arthritics for different reasons. This last group includes the sex hormones, such as oestrogen and testosterone.

THE PITUITARY GLAND

This tiny gland, of only 1cm (less than $\frac{1}{2}$) in diameter, is the master gland of the endocrine system, controlling from deep in its seat in the brain such vital functions as thyroid and sexual function, growth rate and the metabolism of food and water.

It is suspended from the hypothalamus and is intimately connected with it. Together, the two guide the body's unconscious functions (for how the conscious has a bearing on the unconscious for better or worse, see Thymus and Chapter 11).

The pituitary secretes at least ten hormones, of which the best known are possibly GH (growth hormone), FSH and LH (follicle-stimulating hormones, known to all women who have had fertility treatments) and ACTH (adrenocorticotropic hormone), which is known because it was one of the first key hormones to be isolated. It exerts a controlling role over the production of steroids by the adrenal glands and is adversely affected by steroids given artificially for the treatment of rheumatoid arthritis, asthma and some skin diseases. In effect, such steroids, given over a long time permanently depress ACTH production from the pituitary, and the patient becomes dependent on steroid therapy for dealing with stressful experiences, which is another reason for always trying to treat a disease at source, not just trying to alter its effects.

The pituitary has a controlling influence in the biorhythms of the body and in particular the menstrual cycle, since it releases the hormones that stimulate ovulation.

All the endocrine glands interdepend on each other, so if one is not working properly, it is a good indication that the whole system has been thrown out of kilter by persistent stress, poor diet or the taking of a medication or drug, including sleeping pills and tranquillizers, that is interfering with glandular synchronicity. However, this daunting fact has a positive side, in that any effort made with diet or with stress-management, whichever is appropriate, or with discontinuation of an interfering drug will bring about marked improvement. Note: the discontinuation of steroids must be very carefully monitored by your medical advisor, as with all drugs which have induced dependency.

THE THYROID GLAND

There was a time, at the turn of this century, when goitre (the swelling of the thyroid gland in the neck) was a commonly seen reaction of the gland enlarging in its attempts to cope with iodine deficiency in the diet. Pop-eyes always suggest that an over-active thyroid may be present. Nowadays, iodine is added to domestic salt, so the deficiency seldom occurs.

The bi-lobed thyroid gland found in the neck just below the larynx, is the regulator of body metabolism. Those who have warm, moist skin, a good appetite and who bound out of bed in the mornings, are unlikely to have thyroid deficiency. Those who have very low blood pressure, feel the cold terribly, whose voices have a tendency to get husky and hoarse and whose hair is noticeably thinning on the outer third of their eyebrows, may be on the way to one. Since the amount of energy we have at our disposal is regulated by the thyroid, as is weight control, it is worth having thyroid levels checked if there are signs of excess in either group of symptoms such as are described above.

In addition to controlling metabolic rate, the thyroid also plays a key role in the control of calcium levels in the blood. Nerve function and muscular response depend on stable calcium levels in the blood, and bone structure may be altered as a result in changes in it, too. When these go awry, calcium can be laid down in the wrong places, such as the walls of the blood vessels, or taken out of vital tissues, including the bones. So important is this that calcium intake must always be monitored, especially after middle age. It is terribly important to have the mineral levels of the body checked through simple hair analysis at least once a year, whatever your age, since the minerals interrelate with each other.

THE PARATHYROIDS

Four of these tiny glands sit on the thyroid gland, and these are also responsible for control of calcium levels. They release hormones that mobilize, conserve and prevent calcium loss, and they work in synchrony with the thyroid-releasing (calcitonin) hormone, which lowers blood calcium. The two are in constant interplay, because the equilibrium of any environmentally responsive system is achieved only by action, not stagnation. The world is always changing, our needs are always changing, and the body has to adapt to this.

Vitamin D is very important for this part of the endocrine function to work. People who do not get enough from sunlight must take a supplement containing it. Because more and more of our lives are spent indoors it seems wise, if we live in the northern hemisphere, to take a supplement anyway. In addition, living under full-spectrum lighting will help solve another problem connected with SAD (seasonal affective disorder; see below) as well.

THE ADRENAL GLANDS

These two vital glands, which sit above the kidneys, are intimately involved with the body's reaction to stress. They are also involved with key metabolic functions such as glucose metabolism. Adrenal hormones also maintain the vital-for-health electrolyte balance of the body by juggling the levels of the current-conveying minerals, potassium and sodium. It is useful to remember that the body works on a delicate form of electricity, which functions through the offices of the minerals we ingest, and that this function depends on the maintenance of critical levels of certain minerals. Eating too much salt (sodium), which modern diets encourage, interferes with this balance, so we should try to eat more potassium, which is found in fruits, especially bananas, and eat less salt. See Chapter 10 for more information about necessary salt levels and so forth.

WATER PILLS AND THE ADRENAL GLANDS

Another habit which causes upsets in the potassium/sodium balance is taking diuretics (water pills) over a long period of time. These cause potassium to be lost from the body, and unless an adequate potassium supplement is taken with them, they can have long-term damaging effects, possibly just as unfriendly to health as that of the initial condition for which they were given! Another example of why symptoms must be traced back to source and treated there.

BETA-BLOCKERS

Beta-blockers also work on certain aspects of adrenal function, blocking, as their name suggests, certain messages conveyed by the hormones from getting through. The action of all hormones released by the endocrine system is something like that of a bunch of keys, each of which will fit only one lock to 'open the door' to a series of effects. It is not always possible to single out the one effect needed without eliciting a lot of other unwanted side effects.

In life-threatening conditions there is not much else that can be done but give such drugs, but these drugs could better be viewed as buying time for the patient who can then begin a total review of his or her lifestyle, eating habits and so on. The recovery of the body, even from advanced disease conditions, is little short of miraculous.

SEX HORMONES AND THE ADRENALS
There are one other group of hormones produced by the busy adrenals which seem to be of minor importance and that is the sex hormones. Far more are produced in the ovaries and testes, but these probably come into play under certain circumstances. For example, it is known that a small percentage of lucky women undergo an easy menopause with few after-effects because their adrenal glands take over production of sufficient oestrogen to keep them symptom-free. Preserving the healthy function of one's adrenal glands could have other benefits reaped in the second part of life.

THE THYMUS GLAND
Situated just behind the sternum or breast bone, this gland has received a lot of publicity lately because of the T-cells it produces. All AIDS sufferers lack these vital cells, which are part of the body's complex immune system. The thymus and it functions have only recently been fathomed. For a long time it was thought that the gland was active during childhood and adolescence but after that it atrophied. In fact it is uniquely concerned with the immune function and as such will be discussed in Chapter 11.

THE PINEAL GLAND
The pineal is another gland whose function was not thought to be of significance until recently. Situated deep in the brain behind the hypothalamus, it appears to be linked to the eyes and to be sensitive to night/day (circadian) rhythms.

Most people have heard of SAD (Seasonal Affective Disorder), which affects an increasing number of people, causing them to be sluggish and both mentally and sexually unresponsive, even depressed, during the winter months. There is also a tendency to crave carbohydrates; in fact the whole syndrome resembles a type of hibernation.

It has now been posited that our increasingly indoor lifestyles, more and more established in this century, cause an excess of a hormone-like substance called melatonin to build up in our bodies. This substance, probably originating in the pineal gland, induces a mental sluggishness appropriate for night time and sleep. It is produced during darkness and is dispelled in truly bright light. However, even fluorescent light, such as is found in a brightly-lit kitchen or office, is only equal to poor twilight. So in winter months and in non-sunny climates, critical limits of melatonin may persist in some which are not dispensed in dark mornings. SAD does not occur in summer or in tropical climes.

The fact that the SAD syndrome is readily and quickly controlled by exposure to bright sunlight or its substitute, full-spectrum lighting, indicates that light is the vital factor involved. Our own electric lights do not give out the full band of light needed to dispense melatonin; however, specially constructed, full-spectrum lights, both fluorescent and otherwise, can and do mimic sunlight, so it seems wise to at least incorporate one such light in the family room of every household (see Useful Addresses for suppliers).

It is postulated that the effect of melatonin affects the reproductive cycle and indeed all biorhythms. When such a simple solution is at hand, it seems foolish not to take precautionary measures.

Interestingly, the pineal gland has always been associated with the esoteric concept of the third eye. Findings suggest that the pineal gland was indeed the evolutionary precursor to the modern eye.

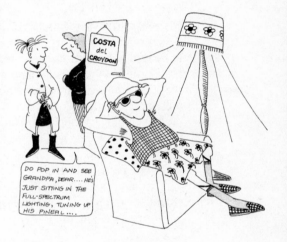

SEMI-ENDOCRINE GLANDS

The pancreas and kidneys are both organs and part of the endocrine system. Each secretes hormones as well as performing their organic functions. The stomach also secretes hormones, which alter both its gastric solutions and the actual movements.

The pancreas secretes the well-known hormone insulin. Inside the pancreas, which also secretes digestive juices directly into the duodenum, are some million ovoid structures, the Islets of Langerhans. These are not more than a hundred millionths of a metre in diameter, yet they are responsible for controlling one of the key metabolic processes of the body – glucose metabolism. Without insulin sugar diabetes occurs, which used to be fatal but is now kept under control by the artificial injection of insulin into the bloodstream. Once thought to be an irreversible condition, mild diabetes can now be controlled by diet. Like any other organ in the body, the pancreas will re-invigorate itself under a programme of the right diet, and cell-building programmes such as those described in Chapter 11.

The pancreas stretches across the upper abdomen at about waist level. Its functions are further described in Chapter 4, since the enzymes it produces play a key role in the digestion of food.

The kidneys (see Chapter 10) also produce hormones that control and exert influence on blood pressure and on the vital formation of red blood cells in the bone marrow. The workings of the body are a marvel of interdependency; no one part can ever be isolated and viewed as an entity in its own right.

THE SEX GLANDS

No other part of the body arouses such preoccupation as that part which makes us either male or female. But although an embryo's sex is determined at fertilization, the potential for development of either male or female gonads is still present, and it is not until after the eighth week of pregnancy that the embryo reveals the secret of what its sex will be. Although male and female sex organs seem vastly different, they do have biological origins in common. Thus there are correspondences between the ovaries and the testes, the labia and the scrotum, and the clitoris and the penis. However, their common beginnings soon become divergent paths that lead to the opposite poles of male and female expression of life. These differences begin with biological diversities but extend to mental, behavioural and psychological parameters as well. Yet throughout life, there is something of the female in every male and vice versa.

THE MALE GONADS
The primary sex organs of the male are the penis, which transfers the male seed or spermatozoa to the vagina of the female, and two testes, in which the sperm are formed. Other parts of the system include the muscular tube, the vas deferens, which links the testes to the urethra in the penis, in which the sperm are matured and from which they are propelled in ejaculation, and the prostate gland, seminal vesicles and bulbo-urethral glands, all three of which add their separate secretions to sperm to ultimately comprise 90 per cent of the seminal fluid.

THE TESTES
The construction of each testis bears tribute to the body's fantastic ability to pack a macrocosm into a microcosm, for there are no fewer than 200 tightly coiled sperm-producing tubules in each testis, each one of which is about 60cm (2ft) long! These in turn lead into the beginning

of the vas deferens, a highly-convoluted duct called the epididymus, whose very name suggests its labyrinthine nature, for if its folds were to be unravelled they would stretch to nearly 6 metres (20 feet). When it is considered that no fewer than 3 million spermatozoa are produced for each and every ejaculation, then the tremendous scope and magnitude of testicular production of sperm is understood.

However, the true endocrine activity of the testes is not the sperm-producing activity, which is their secretion, but the formation of the male hormone testosterone, which is released, as are all hormones, directly into the bloodstream. It is under this influence that testicular activity originates and is conducted through life.

Although some testosterone is produced even in the foetus and throughout childhood, it is not until puberty that the sex glands become active and cause the secondary sex characteristics we have come to associate with being male to develop – the voice deepens, because of the effect of testosterone on the larynx; pubic, axillary and facial hair develops; there is a tremendous increase in muscle and skeleton mass (testosterone is an anabolic steroid, which means that it builds up the body); the sebaceous glands beneath the surface of the skin increase their activity (which can lead to acne at first); and there are also certain other accompanying personality changes, including the increased agression and boisterousness associated with male personality and the male sex drive.

After that production of sperm continues until old age. Most experts recognize that there is a male menopause – a falling off of both hormone and sperm production around about the age of fifty – but it has nothing of the finality of the female menopause at about the same age, during which egg production, the female equivalent of sperm production, ceases altogether, although sex drive does not, because in both female and male this is thought to be regulated by testosterone, which is produced by females in the adrenal glands. The testes also produce the female hormone oestrogen in minute quantities.

VIVE LA DIFFERENCE!

Although testosterone production varies slightly over a 24-hour period, its production follows a steady pattern showing none of the cyclical swings to which the female cycle is subject. Thus, the nature of the male is more likely to remain on an even keel. There is no doubt that hormones and their presence or absence have a tremendous effect on personality, and to know this is to acknowledge a key factor in our lives; both in respect of the sex urges of the male, which are more urgent, more consistent and differently expressed from those of the cyclically-governed female, and in respect of the resultant personality divergences.

TESTES AND TEMPERATURE

It is interesting to note that body construction is very wise in positioning the testes in the scrotum, outside the body cavity. This is because for ideal sperm production the temperature must remain about 2 degrees cooler than the rest of the body. Men who wear tight underclothing or do anything that combats nature's wisdom in this matter often have a lower sperm count, which can be an infertility factor in some cases. The use of cotton underwear can make all the difference, since it is absorbent and allows heat to disperse.

ERECTION AND EJACULATION

Erection of the penis is due to arterial dilation of its spongy tissues coupled with compression of the veins which would normally allow the blood to flow out of the penis and back to the heart. The whole process is controlled by the autonomic (involuntary and not under conscious control) nervous system. The procedure is, therefore, very susceptible to stress, as every man knows! Furthermore, a mixture of sympathetic (constriction) and parasympathetic (dilation and relaxation) activity is at work, one branch being responsible for one effect, and one the opposite (read about this in Chapter 7). The whole activity is a tribute to the power of the hormones governing the sex drive in that most times the system works without a hitch!

Ejaculation is a reflex peristaltic contraction of the vas deferens and seminal vesicles, an activity similar to the muscular propulsions in the gut, but much more powerful.

PROBLEMS OF SEXUAL FUNCTION

Fortunately there is not much physically that can go wrong with sperm production. However, functional problems are legion, and they include impotence and premature ejaculation, which come into the realm of psychosexual problems, since they are nearly always of emotional origin. Because nearly all parental, social and religious conditioning about sex and the sexual organs is negative ('don't do this ... don't do that ... this is disgusting ... that is simply not done'), it is hardly surprising that we are left with an inheritance of guilt, remorse and shame, and very often little or no conscious understanding of how to put it right.

There are organizations specializing in psychosexual counselling, and access is possible through one's doctor, or, if this constitutes an unwelcome area of enquiry, from VD clinics (where every query is treated anonymously) and most local councils. The telephone book is a good source of such information.

CONTROLLING PREMATURE EJACULATION

Sex experts Masters and Johnson devised a technique that is now recognized as helpful for managing this common and curable problem, especially with young males. In this the female brings the male nearly to orgasm and then prevents orgasm by briefly compressing the penis between her fingers just below the head. Masters and Johnson believed that once the couple come to realize that in this way premature ejaculation can easily be prevented, their anxiety disappears, and ultimately they can achieve normal coitus without resorting to this squeeze technique.

IMPOTENCE

This is nearly always psychogenic in males under the age of 40. Fear of being impotent frequently causes impotence, and so the poor male is caught in a self-perpetuating problem. Because the erection reaction is part of the nervous system response, which is not under conscious control, the problem is usually deep-seated and may have to do with unconscious feelings of inadequacy, hostility, fear or guilt, all or any of which have been engendered during childhood or adolescence. Ejaculatory impotence (inability to ejaculate in intercourse) is nearly always psychogenic in origin and is often associated with ideas of contamination or with memories of traumatic experiences.

Attaching blame to the cause of these problems is pointless. Instead it is better to unearth the origin of the cause, buried deep in the unconscious. This can be reached but one needs a sensitive guide on the journey. Networks of psychotherapists and counsellors such as the British Association for Counselling, or the UK Standing Conference for Psychotherapy, or the Westminster Pastoral Foundation, or the British Association for Counselling, can provide qualified and sensitive help (see Useful Addresses).

PROSTATE PROBLEMS

This gland, and its tendency to become inflamed or enlarged, is one of the more common sites of physical problems, especially for older men. However, difficulties may be averted by some simple remedies and avoidances.

Most experts agree that problems of this nature can be exacerbated by sexual excitation without ejaculation, since the prostate becomes engorged with fluids for the ejaculate without the release of them. Developing sexual regularity is also advised.

Walking is such good exercise, not only for the prostate but for the whole body. Sitz baths, in which the scrotum is immersed for a few minutes in cold water, also provide tone, but sitz baths of very warm water to which camomile tea has been added should be favoured if there is an acute condition or inflammation.

Dietary advice suggests the taking of pollen, pumpkin or sunflower seeds, almonds (not salted or roasted) and vitamins E and F (essential fatty acids) plus a multi-vitamin mineral supplement rich in zinc.

Looking after the prostate makes good sense because it is one of the commonest sites of cancer in later life and one of the most difficult to treat.

THE FEMALE GONADS

The sex glands of the female are the two ovaries, and all other sexual organs are subsidiary to their function. In a young girl they contain some 700,000 egg-producing follicles, but most of these atrophy before or just after puberty.

Three hormones are produced by the ovaries – oestrogen, which is the feminizing hormone, progesterone, which is the hormone that comes on line during the second half of the menstrual cycle to prepare the uterus for receiving the egg, and relaxin, which is produced only during the last stages of pregnancy (see below).

Two uterine tubes conduct ova (eggs) from the ovaries to the uterus, the funnel-ended fallopian tubes. Other parts of the female reproductive system are, of course, the uterus, which is shaped like an inverted pear, and under non-pregnant conditions is about 7.5cm (3in) long and weighs a mere 28g (1oz); in full-term pregnancy this increases to an amazing 30cm (12in) long and weighs, apart from the baby, 1kg (2.6lb).

The bottom of the uterus is button-shaped, and it is known as the cervix, a muscular opening which connects with the vagina. Vagina means sheath, and under normal conditions this sheath or access to the womb is angled backwards so that in fact the uterus lies at right angles to it (anteverted).

The female external genitalia include the structures placed around the entrance to the vagina, and they are the fatty-tissued mons, which lies in front of the pubic bone, the labia majora (outer lips) and labia minora (inner lips). At the top of the labia minora is the clitoris, which is of erectile tissue similar to the penis. In between the clitoris and the vaginal opening is the opening to the bladder, the urethra. When it is additionally considered that the anus, or opening to the bowel, lies just behind the vagina, the extreme importance of feminine hygiene becomes even more apparent.

The feminine (menstrual) cycle, which usually begins at around the ages of 11 to 13, although it may be as late as 16, is marked by period-icity. This in turn is marked by understandable fluctuations in emotions. Hormones are powerful substances, and it is the lucky female who can manage to keep on an even monthly keel despite them. Recognizing this instead of denying it is of key importance in controlling the boundaries of the swings, either by diet (see PMT) or by mental control.

THE MENSTRUAL CYCLE

This is not so much a curse of nature as a wonder of it. The lining of the uterus must be prepared to a critical level of perfection for pregnancy, and the body anticipates this every month. Each month a fresh lining is prepared for the egg, and this involves the action of several hormones, all controlled by the pituitary gland. Also each month one ovarian follicle ripens under the stimulation of the follicle-releasing hormone (FSH) of the pituitary. The fertility drug mimics this influence, but it is not known how nature limits its stimulation to the preparation of one egg, while the drug stimulates multiple eggs and results in multiple births.

During the 14th day of the cycle, luteinizing hormone (LH) is released from the pituitary and causes the follicle to rupture and release the egg into the fallopian tube, where it is propelled along by numerous small hairs, which allow the egg to move in only one direction.

As soon as this occurs a second hormone, progesterone, comes on line to further prepare the lining of the womb to receive the egg. Progesterone is an anabolic steroid and it causes an increase in body metabolism, with a corresponding rise in temperature. This rise is useful in detecting whether ovulation has occurred, and it is used for this purpose, and also for contraceptive purposes for those following the rhythm method, for they know that the four to five day danger period has begun.

If the egg is not fertilized the lining of the uterus breaks down and is sloughed off approximately two weeks later and menstruation occurs.

THE SIGNIFICANCE OF MENSTRUATION

Although they may be superficially annoyed by the menstrual cycle, its absence upsets women of child-bearing age far more, for whatever reasons. While most women think they are controlling the menstrual cycle, by taking the pill to avoid pregnancy or by denying and masking its effects in a society that now expects them to carry on as if nothing is happening, it is, in fact, controlling them at a far deeper level, although some feminists would like to deny this.

This is partly due to the fact that disturbances of the menstrual cycle are often present in illness and at times of severe emotional stress. Thus the return of the cycle somehow indicates that all is well again. It is reassuring to know in this context that, important though the menstrual cycle may be, it is not essential for good health. It is simply that as a reproductive and sexual function, it has deep-seated significance. Amenorrhoea (lack of periods) should always be investigated, not only for this reason but also because underlying physical conditions may indicate the presence of disease. A welcome exception to this is after pregnancy, when a breast-feeding mother may not have a period until she stops breast-feeding, which is nature's way of protecting her from an early recurrence of pregnancy before her body is ready. This is not infallible, however.

PRE-MENSTRUAL TENSION (PMT OR PMS)

Most women suffer from this to a greater or lesser degree at some stage, and it is one of the commonest debilitating afflictions which already burdened young women and their families have to suffer – and its effects seem to increase with age, and with the number of children born.

Yet it can be simply controlled with a combination of nutritional therapy and diet. PMT is really a sign that the body is not functioning as well as it can. Under perfect conditions it could probably be eliminated altogether; under the stressful and polluted conditions of 20th-century life, the most we hope for is to keep it to levels at which it does not affect well-being or vital relationships.

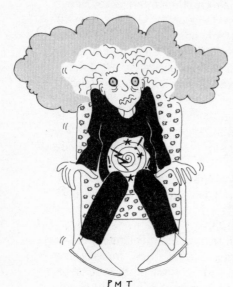

PMT

Experts, such as the well-known researcher Dr Guy Abraham from California, have identified several types of PMT, which need marginally different approaches.

● PMT-A: anxiety, nervous tension, mood swings, irritability.

● PMT-H: hormonal weight gain, bloating, swelling, breast tenderness.

● PMT-C: craving for specific foods and sweets, headaches, tiredness, heart-pounding, dizziness, fainting.

● PMT-D: depression, forgetfulness, crying spells, confusion, sleeplessness.

● PMT-A sufferers appeared to be lacking in vitamin B_6 and magnesium. PMT-H was the most complex type; again vitamin B_6 and magnesium were lacking, but there were also stress factors, which had to be addressed with counselling, plus a craving for sugar, which suggested dietary imbalances and in some cases allergies. PMT-C demonstrated specific deficiencies of nutrients such as essential fatty acids. PMT-D sufferers often had environmental factors to consider, as well as dietary imbalances and certain vitamin and mineral insufficiencies.

Dr Abraham devised a nutritional supplement, Optivite, which goes a long way to help most PMT sufferers. There is nothing mysterious about it, simply that its vitamins and minerals are arranged in such a way that they specifically serve PMT sufferers with dosages scaled so that the six tablets most women needed to take – three at breakfast, three at lunch – did not prove nutritionally excessive. Some women safely take more. PMT-C is also helped by taking evening primrose oil.

In addition to nutritional supplementation, which suggests that yet again modern 'processed' diets are a contributory cause of many health conditions, it was also advocated that all foods eaten should be reviewed, with foods that were craved being kept to a minimum, if eaten at all. This is because foods that are craved are frequently foods to which one is allergic. Later, when the nutritional supplementation has alleviated the symptoms, these foods may be acceptable, but most young women feel so well on their new diet that they not only stay on it themselves but also change their family over to it.

Dietary advice suggests cutting out the following: sweets, chocolates, refined carbohydrates, fried and fatty foods, carbonated drinks, salty foods, tea, coffee and alcohol. There is a definite link between coffee drinking and sore breasts. Sufferers are also advised to eat plenty of leafy green vegetables and salad, wholefoods, such as unprocessed grains and cereals, lean meat, poultry, and in particular fish containing essential oils, such as herring, halibut and salmon (especially for breast tenderness). The Women's Nutritional Advisory Service in the UK performs a very reasonably priced advice service specifically tailored to the individual (see Useful Addresses).

Most women are delighted with their progress after three months – six in severe cases – and so are their husbands and children!

PREGNANCY AND HEALTH

Most nutritionists agree that preparing for a baby should begin long before its conception with the eating of good, healthy food such as that advocated in Chapter 4, to prepare the body for its task.

Since every mother wants a healthy baby, this seems wise – if you know about your intention! It is also wise not to stress the body by having children too quickly – the two-year gap between births is not just some ideal dreamed up by sociologists, for within that period birth defects increase.

Pregnancy is one of the most medically monitored of healthy states, and most women will be reasonably well looked after and informed during their pre-natal care and visits to the doctor, and indeed most want to find out as much as they can on the subject, realizing what is at stake.

The advice given here pertains to maintaining good health, which means, among other things, not putting on more weight than is recommended. When you consider that the heart must do 25 per cent more work during some states of pregnancy and that the blood supply it must pump also increases by 25 per cent, this alone militates against giving it even more work to do by literally eating for two!

That said, the intake of vital minerals such as calcium, iron and phosphorus must be increased, or minerals will be leached from the mother's system. Pregnancy is an excellent time to seek advice from a nutritional and dietary expert, as there is less scope for getting away with dietary mistakes.

The digestion of pregnant women is weaker than at other times. Because acid production in the stomach decreases, a narrower range of foods can be eaten, and there is all the more reason, therefore, to take a good nutritional and mineral supplement and, possibly, to keep on hand some digestive enzymes such as pineapple bromelain or papaya extract, which are natural aids to digestion and therefore quite safe to take with meals. Peppermint essence – dissolve 5 drops in a small glass of hot water – can be helpful too.

Resting is also of vital importance, as is walking as opposed to standing. During pregnancy the body gains an amazing 3.5–4.5 litres (6–8 pints) of fluid, which explains the swollen lower extremities of later pregnancy. Gentle massage from the feet up to the thighs will help to disperse fluid that is trapped in the legs due to pressure on lymph glands in the pelvic area.

CHILDBIRTH OPTIONS
Examining various ways of giving birth is becoming increasingly popular. Modern medicine, in the interests of safety, has taken over childbirth and has interfered with its natural expressions and rhythms such as naturally occurring birth-times, sometimes to the detriment of the length and difficulty of labour.

It is as well to read modern thought on this matter such as is expressed in books written by Frederick Leboyer and Michel Odent. Facilities for such natural births are increasingly available, but help must be available for any mother who needs medical support should things not go according to plan.

BREAST-FEEDING BONUSES
Breast-feeding deserves a mention since it is good for the baby, which means it is good for the mother, who will have a healthier child. Not only is breast milk perfectly designed for human babies, while all other substitutes may be allergy-forming or indigestible, but it is also now

known that immunity to many diseases is passed with breast milk. Breast milk enables the baby's delicate intestines to be cultivated with a healthy balance of intestinal flora. Research shows that adults who have been breast fed do not suffer to the same extent from disorders of the bowel.

Just before the baby is due, the third ovarian hormone is released into the blood. Called relaxin, this has the effect of loosening the connective tissue between the sacral joints and the pelvis to facilitate the stretching that must occur at birth. Unfortunately, this also is one of the causes of the backache frequently experienced in late pregnancy.

The vulnerable state of the spine under these conditions makes it important not to overdo things or to carry too much in the last few weeks. Also try to arrange the sort of labour that will best serve the back. Squatting to give birth is one of the most natural and safe methods, since it employs the use of gravity and not abuse of muscles!

In the final analysis, one has to accept the conditions imposed by the combination of one's own health, the baby's health and the circumstances available. If these change during labour, it should not be viewed as a sign of failure on the part of the mother to deliver her baby in the desired manner. There is always another time!

AVOIDING PREGNANCY

Since 1960, when the US Food and Drug Administration approved the pill, 150 million women worldwide have used oral contraceptives. Whatever else is said about it, for and against, the pill has transformed the lives of women. It has emancipated them in a way that Emmeline Pankhurst never dreamed possible. The constant monthly fear of becoming pregnant, with all the responsibility, sometimes life-changing, that that entails, became a thing of the past.

A price had to be paid for this, and it was paid by those women who were not compatible with the pill. Nowadays, there are so many versions of it and the incompatible women have been so clearly defined that the risks are minimal, and these always have to be weighed against the health-draining, stress-inducing risk of having unwanted children.

However, the long-term effects of the pill on female health are still unknown. Surprisingly HRT (Hormone Replacement Therapy), which is still viewed with suspicion by some doctors, has a longer track record to support it than the pill. Until more is known, decisions about taking the pill will have to be viewed according to existing factors, including the all important non-physical ones, such as peace of mind, financial and family planning, security of relationship and so on. The long-term effects of disregarding factors such as these could prove far more deleterious to the health of mother and child than the slight risk of taking the pill.

There are books available (*The Pill Protection Plan* – published by Grapevine – is one) that will give future users much more information, nutritional and historical, than will be proffered while the prescription is being written, when only general guidelines can be considered. Again, it is a question of the individual taking responsibility for noting any symptoms and side-effects and acquiring the knowledge that may help both self and experts to make the right choice of pill or to stop taking it altogether.

Here are some of the symptoms which suggest that the pill may be causing side-effects and needs to be changed for another type: acne, allergies, appetite increase, breast tenderness, brittle nails, elevated cholesterol level, depression, hair thinning, headaches, nausea and thrush or urinary tract infections.

Many of these conditions can be adjusted by taking a pill containing a different balance of hormones from the one that is causing the symptoms.

NUTRITION AND THE PILL

Since taking the pill depletes the body's zinc supply and elevates the body's copper levels, which renders it further zinc-deficient, since copper is antagonistic to zinc, taking a supplement of 30mg zinc seems an advisable precaution. Zinc should be taken on its own, apart from other vitamins. Since the pill also affects the status of other vitamins and minerals, a hair analysis six months of so after beginning to take the pill is advised, so that the results can be assessed by an expert and nutritional support may be designed.

One thing the pill will not do is protect its taker against AIDS or any other form of VD. For this a condom is needed, and the female condom has just become available.

Other forms of contraception, such as the IUD (intra-uterine device), the cap and spermicidal jellies, all have their devotees. It is important to know the percentage of safety of each method, information that is available from most clinics who screen women. You should also be aware that the strings of the IUD can get infected, so any sign of discharge or repeated minor infection should not be neglected.

CYSTITIS AND THRUSH

For both of these common 'female' conditions, the main message is to avoid taking antibiotics if you can. Thrush is very often caused by antibiotics, and cystitis is very rarely cured by them, although the original pain and inflammation may subside, leading you to believe that it is. Antibiotics are still handed out willy-nilly for colds and so-called 'flu', for which their effect is questionable anyway, unless or until the complication of a chest infection sets in.

Antibiotics upset the delicate balance of intestinal flora in the gut and can cause far more harm in the long run than the condition for which they were taken (see Chapter 4). Always eat live yoghurt when taking antibiotics or, better still, take a course of antifungals such as nystatin. Do not be silly and let yourself become really ill, but try to avoid them if you can.

CYSTITIS: ALL TOO COMMON CONDITION

Pain, frequency of urination, burning (and ultimately blood) when passing urine is caused by unwanted bugs getting into the urinary tract either during intercourse or from the bowel because of inadequate hygiene.

Experts such as Angela Kilmartin, who has written four books on cystitis and ran a counselling service in the 1970s when the condition was much less understood, advise measures that centre on improved feminine hygiene, since the infecting bacteria usually come from the bowel. Kilmartin recommends this procedure after bowel movements.

Wipe away from, not towards, the uretho/vaginal area. Then, while still seated, take a bottle of water and sluice down with it, using the free hand, not a towel or flannel, to help the cleansing job. Pat dry with paper. The man's hygiene techniques, especially if he is uncircumcised, must also be reviewed. There is no longer any doubt that the incidence of infections in the vaginal area is four times as high through intercourse with uncircumcised men.

Kilmartin also gives the following advice when cystitis is coming on and you are at the frequency/sensitivity stage.

1. Take a urine specimen for later analysis.
2. Drink half a pint of water immediately and repeat every 20 minutes for 3 hours. With the first drink take 2 strong painkillers. Water can be flavoured with weak squash; barley water is good, but plain water is best.
3. Unless you a have a heart condition, on the hour, every hour for 3 hours, take a level teaspoon of bicarbonate of soda in a little water.
4. Fill two hot water bottles. Put one on your back and the other between your legs. This makes the urine feel cooler when it emerges.
5. Once an hour for the 3 hours, drink a coffee cup of strong coffee to help the liquid you are drinking pass out.
6. Do not attempt to go anywhere or do anything: you are fighting a bug. Get a book, lie down and keep warm.

True cystitis will abate in this time, although you should continue to drink a lot for several more hours. If the symptoms do not abate go to the doctor.

THRUSH

Thrush is becoming more and more common as modern dietary habits play havoc with our intestinal flora. There may be more to it than just the itching and milky-looking discharge in the vaginal area, which is (initially anyway) cleared up by creams and pessaries. Read about its more serious forms in Chapter 4. Meanwhile, repeated vaginal attacks should prompt a change in the following habits:

1. Eat and drink fewer sugary things, especially yeast-based things such as beers and wines.
2. Change your underwear to cotton and cut the gussets out of your tights.
3. Do not take antibiotics without taking antifungal pessaries at the same time.
4. Do not sit all day on the edge of office chairs; do not stay in hot baths; do not swim in chlorinated pools without showering and washing after and changing from tight swimsuits.
5. Consider changing your contraceptive pill, and if that does not work, give it up to see if it is the culprit.
6. Review your diet according to suggestions in Chapter 4.

VENEREAL DISEASE AND HEALTH

There are many different kinds of venereal disease, but they have one thing in common; they do not get better by themselves. They are easily cured in the early stages but not later. This also applies to AIDS, which is not invariably fatal.

Here are some details about VD clinics you may or may not know:

● VD clinics are not only free, they treat you anonymously. You do not have to give them any personal details whatsoever.

● VD clinics will usually see you very quickly, but like all medical units they are busy and may be off-putting on the phone. Sometimes it is better just to walk in.

● They are not just for VD but for any kind of infection in the genital area.

● They are usually staffed by non-judgmental people who have seen things far worse than you are likely to present to them.

● They are only interested in stopping the spread of VD and genital infections, not stopping your sex life.

● They segregate the sexes, so you don't have to meet your opposite number.

So wear a wig and take a large pair of sunglasses and a copy of *The Times* or whatever you need to hide behind (one wag entered the male clinic to find – he counted them – twelve copies of *The Times* confronting him!).

How much wiser to take precautions to avoid such problems. The female condom is now on sale; the male condom is and always has been readily available. It is much easier to assume this protection as a matter of course when you are with someone new than to get into long discussions of sexual histories. If ever anyone is going to lie, it will be in this context: how could it be otherwise? When beginning a relationship you are trying to create desire, not to kill it stone dead. Although it may be true that sex can never be as good with condoms as it is without them, that (ideal) situation requires the trust of a steady relationship.

SMEARS AND BREAST SCREENING

Our grandmothers suffered in ignorance and silence from some of the worst of the female diseases, cancer of the breast and of the uterus, but at last, in this one small area of medicine, we are actually being encouraged to practice prevention!

The cervical smear, which is uncomfortable but painless, can warn you years ahead of any problem while the condition is readily reversible. Likewise techniques for screening and excising breast lumps are not the disfiguring ones they used to be, provided they are caught early. Let it be said that statistics do not favour breast removal in cases of cancer. Those who have had lumpectomies statistically fare just as well and surgical techniques are improving all the time. Research has also shown that survival depends on a positive attitude as much as on any other factor, together with the necessary changes in diet and lifestyle outlined in Chapter 12 on the Immune System.

HOW TO EXAMINE YOUR BREASTS
It is far better to check your breasts once a month. Do this just after menstruation, because they are less sensitive then and less affected by hormones. Lie down and work gently from the outer and upper quadrants, working with the flat of the hand and extended fingers, not your finger tips. Look for any signs of puckering on the skin's surface,

retraction of the nipples or education from them. Don't expect to feel anything more than pea-sized, but know that a lump will have been growing for some considerable time to have reached pea-size.

Most lumps are benign, but do not delay. Take a trusted woman friend with you – she will remember what you do not because of your fear.

Never accept one opinion or one course of action, especially if you don't like it. Doctors vary enormously about their attitudes to breast treatments, so find out where your local screening clinic is and go and talk to them. Buy books, ring, if desperate, or write to the health editor of well-known magazines and ask for leaflets of latest information. Put a stamped, self-addressed envelope in the post immediately with a reminder note about what you want. This information keeps changing as techniques are constantly updated, so you should always seek the latest publications and information.

INFERTILITY: A REVERSIBLE CONDITION?

Ten per cent of marriages are called barren by the authorities, thus labelling them, by the use of that terrible word, as lacking in some way.

Many couples adjust and actually live less demanding lives without children, but for the few for whom the fulfilment of their relationship rests on having a family, there is a long road ahead, of medical examinations, medicalized sex, interference with hormones and, at the end of the road, the possibility that none of it will work and by that stage that the adoption door might even be closed as well.

There is one avenue that is rarely pursued and that is to make concerted attempts to improve the health of both partners, especially where the cause of infertility is not clear cut. So read the chapters on digestion and elimination, incorporate some form of healthy exercise into the lifestyle and try to reduce levels of that enemy to health, stress. Who knows what might happen?

THE MENOPAUSE AND HRT

Freud said 'Biology is destiny'. For women entering the menopause the truth of that statement becomes poignant, if not painful. It is a peak time for marriage breakdown as women can lose both their self-esteem and, quite unnecessarily, libido because they think they are 'finished' in some way.

It is a time when nebulous symptoms exacerbate any problems

women may be having, such as irritability, tiredness, depression or headaches, all of which can be attributed to many causes until the arrival of the unmistakable symptoms, such as hot flushes or flashes, night sweats and joint pains, proclaim the real cause.

In the UK an estimated 2 million of the 10 million menopausal women suffer severe symptoms in the belief that there is nothing that can be done. There is – but not tranquillizers, which often make it worse.

HRT (hormone replacement therapy) in its modern form has been exonerated from causative links with cancer, with thrombosis and from breakthrough bleeding since adjustments have been made to the types and doses of hormones used.

Furthermore, HRT can actually protect women from that worst of all scourges, osteoporosis, a post-menopausal condition in which as much as 30–40 per cent of calcium gets leached out of the bones making them brittle and likely to break. It is estimated that 9 thousand women a year in the UK die of such complications and 22,000 become permanent invalids.

HRT can also protect women from atheroscleosis, hardening of the arteries – there is a 50 per cent reduction in risk – to say nothing of the cosmetic and feminizing effects of maintaining better skin and muscle tone, alleviating vaginal dryness and so forth.

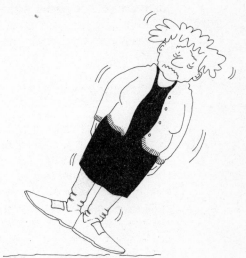

HRT *CAN KEEP YOU ON AN EVEN KEEL* .....

Libido is not affected by the menopause, except psychologically. The response which facilitates arousal and orgasm is orchestrated not by oestrogen, but by small amounts of the male hormone testosterone, which a woman produces. But because oestrogen-deficient symptoms, such as vaginal dryness and soreness, plus debilitating tiredness and indifference, complicate the issue, many women go off sex at the very time when family life allows it to be enjoyed with more leisure.

Only about 10 per cent of UK women are receiving HRT, largely because of the resistance of a medical profession that remembers the scare of the 1970s, when research in the USA, where the treatment is far more popular, linked it with cancer of the uterus. Now a second hormone, progestogen, has been added to the treatment to be sure this does not happen. Yet doctors still cite the risk factor, forgetting the risks of osteoporosis, atheroscleosis, breakdown of the important, sexual aspect of marriage, loss of self-esteem due to ageing, loss of energy and so on.

In the final analysis, it has to be left to women themselves to weigh up the pros and cons, to take a decision, and, if for it, to insist on the treatment, which in the UK is available on the National Health. One book that might be helpful in the pursuit of knowledge is *No Change* by Dr Wendy Cooper.

Some clinics specialize in advising women about HRT. Two in the UK are the Amarant Trust and Marie Stopes (see Useful Addresses). There are also clinics who will scan for osteoporosis and advise suitable preventive measures, which should begin long before the onset of the menopause (see Useful Addresses).

10

*

THE ELIMINATION AND EXCRETORY SYSTEMS

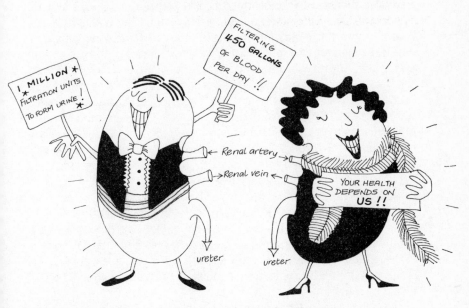

I MILLION FILTRATION UNITS TO FORM URINE!

FILTERING 450 GALLONS OF BLOOD PER DAY!!

Renal artery
Renal vein

YOUR HEALTH DEPENDS ON US!!

ureter

ureter

★ THE STARS OF ELIMINATION ★

IN THIS CHAPTER

✳ Four pillars of health ✳ Five-fold paths of elimination
✳ Heroic kidneys (and bladder) ✳ Understanding urinary
infections ✳ External and internal pollution ✳ Enlivening
lymph and its seven-part network ✳ The wonders of skin
brushing ✳ Aromatherapy and lymph drainage ✳ Diets fit for
detoxification ✳ Skin and how to care for it
✳ Overcoming cellulite ✳ Acne

It is generally agreed that good elimination is one of the four pillars of good health. (The other three are a strong, slow heartbeat, healthy digestion and a positive attitude to life.) If wastes cannot be got rid of, they clog the system. The body, wise in this as in all things, does not just rely on one organ to eliminate waste, but on several, which work in harness and independently.

There are five main elimination systems: the kidneys, the bowels, the skin, the lungs and the lymphatic system. Each has a slightly different way of dealing with the body's waste problems. Some have additional roles besides elimination; one could almost think of them moonlighting!

The lymphatic system, for example, is not involved only in elimination of wastes such as dead cells, but it is also part of the immune system, since it produces antibodies to fight bacterial, fungal and other invaders.

The skin is the largest organ in the body, a miraculous substance which regenerates and repairs itself, is easy to clean, is both absorbent and water-resistant, breathes and stretches to adapt both to our internal state and to the external one, darkens in summer to keep out excess light, pales in winter to let it in . . . if makers of artificial fabrics could reproduce any two or three of skin's attributes they would make a fortune. However, one of skin's chief attributes is its rarely considered elimination function. Through its pores it eliminates both water and solvents which the body no longer needs, such as excess mineral salts, acting as a back-up for the kidneys in this respect.

The lungs take in vital oxygen from the air and facilitate its entry into the bloodstream, but they also eliminate the by-products of respiration, water and carbon dioxide, as well as germs, dust and other impurities breathed in with the air. One of the first-line reactions of the body is to cough, an extremely powerful expulsion reaction (see Chapter 6). So think twice about supressing a cough, at least in the early stages of a cold or allergic reaction.

The bowel eliminates some water and dietary residues, including any microbes which may have entered with food.

Last, but not least, are the stars of elimination, the unsung heroes, about which most people know less than possibly any other part of the body (except perhaps the lymph) and they are the kidneys.

KIDNEYS: STARS OF ELIMINATION

If we may digress for one moment into astrology, the kidneys are said to rule Libra, Sign of the Balance, and the appropriateness of this connection can be seen when it is understood that not only do the kidneys regulate the composition and consistency of blood, eliminating excesses and topping up deficiencies, but they also maintain the balance of fluids in the body to exact requirements.

In this they are the peers of elimination. All other eliminatory organs eliminate without discretion, a bit like waste disposal units or most garbage collectors. What goes in gets eliminated. But the kidneys actually go through the garbage, piece by piece, salvaging what can be recycled and only getting rid of a tiny residue of totally unreusable muck. To do this a huge proportion of the body's recirculating blood supply is shunted through to them, no less than 1,800 litres a day – that's nearly 400 gallons!

The kidneys filter all that blood, and out of it they extract no less than 170–180 litres (37–40 gallons) of water or put another way over 100 1.5 litre bottles of mineral water! Line them up in your mind's eye and consider this Herculean task.

The story doesn't end there: they then reabsorb all but on average 1.5 litres (3 pints) of it, concentrating all the poisons, casts, unwanted salts and end-products of body metabolism into roughly that amount of urine, to be expelled in the course of a day.

More than any other body system they are responsible for homoeostasis, a word that has come to represent stability of the body – health in other words. From their central position in the small of the back, one each side of the spine, these two bean-shaped organs battle to keep us in balance.

Nature has carefully provided us with two kidneys in order to perform these key functions, but we can do with one at a pinch – in fact, one in 500 people is born without a second kidney, to say nothing of all those walking around with single kidney transplants!

THE INNER SEA OF LIFE
The kidney has evolved to enable us to live on dry land and not in the sea. To do this water and salts must be conserved and wastes eliminated in a concentrated form. Our internal sea must be kept both pure and minerally consistent. Despite vagaries of diet, tissue fluids have to be strictly regulated as to volume, chemical composition and osmotic pressure in order to facilitate the two-way exchanges needed for cellular metabolism.

KIDNEY FUNCTION
Kidneys are really filtration units. The units of filtration are called nephrons of which there are about 1 million. Blood enters the kidneys via the renal artery, which subdivides into tufts of tiny capillaries called glomeruli. The structure of each glomerulus further intensifies the arterial pressure of the blood, so that it gets spun out or separated, the larger red corpuscles remaining in the arteries, while water and salts (plasma)

pass out into the receiving capsule of the nephron, called Bowman's capsule.

From there, the liquid, which will ultimately become urine, embarks on a journey around an infinite number of hairpin-bend tubules, during which two-way exchanges take place between closely entwined blood capillaries and the filtrate. The end-result is that the larger molecules of protein and glucose remain in the blood, while waste products such as ammonia and creatinine, which gives urine its characteristic odour, remain in the tubules and eventually pass into the ureter and collect in the bladder.

As this filtrate traverses the tubules, it becomes concentrated in the major hairpin bend, the loop of Henle. Here, most of the water and salts are reabsorbed, leaving just the small amount that will become urine. This process of forcing liquids at pressure through such fine networks of tubules takes an enormous amount of energy – in fact, about one-eighth of the total energy used by a resting person is appropriated to kidney function.

Obviously, the whole process depends on pressure, and although the kidneys can regulate their internal circulation, they have great difficulty in doing so if blood pressure is extremely high or extremely low. High blood pressure is more common than low blood pressure, and that is why concern is always felt about the effects of high blood pressure on kidney function.

THE URINARY BLADDER AND URETHRAL TUBES

These form a vital part of the body's main excretory system. All excretory systems have to have contact with the outside environment, and in so doing they are vulnerable to infection from outside. Thus urinary tract infections are quite common, especially in women because their urethra is extremely short, 3–4cm (1¼–1½in) compared with that of men, which is about 20cm (8in) long.

The bladder itself is a hollow, three-layered organ of variable capacity with a powerful muscle coat that empties the organ when it contracts, and two muscular sphincters – one at the base of the bladder and one at the opening of the urethra – which keep the exit closed at other times. Nerves arising from the bladder send information to both conscious and unconscious parts of the brain about its fullness – the fuller it gets the more messages are received.

When the bladder empties, it is a symphony of muscular coordination between voluntary and involuntary groups. As the powerful bladder muscle contracts, the sphincter muscles relax, the muscles of the abdominal wall contract, to increase pressure on the bladder, the diaphragm descends, and breath is usually held, while the muscles on the floor of the abdomen relax! Whew!

A normal bladder empties its contents completely and this is important because any urine left behind would tend to become stagnant.

In design and urinary function, men definitely score over women. Quite apart from the protective advantage of the extra length of urethra, they also have a safety margin built into sphincter design: if something goes wrong with their internal sphincter, they can still maintain continence with the outer sphincter, whereas a woman cannot. It is all the more important for her to exercise the muscles of the pelvic floor by contracting and relaxing the urethral sphincter a dozen or so times a day. This should be part of any exercise programme, and can be done while you are waiting for a bus, waiting in a supermarket queue or whatever – giving purpose to one of life's most annoying aspects, the waiting game.

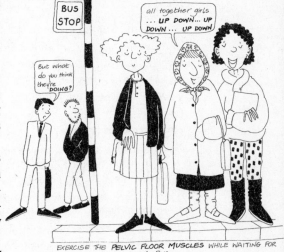

EXERCISE THE **PELVIC FLOOR MUSCLES** WHILE WAITING FOR A BUS....

COMMON INFECTIONS OF THE URINARY TRACT

The above-described anatomical differences between men and women are responsible for cystitis being far more common in women than it is in men.

Cystitis, and how to control it, is discussed in Chapter 9, but it is worth mentioning that the practice of passing urine after intercourse can protect, since it flushes out the urinary tract.

A more sinister form of urinary tract infection is NSU, non-specific urethritis. This, like any infection in this area, should never be neglected as infections can pass upwards, progressively affecting the bladder and ultimately the kidneys.

OEDEMA (FLUID IN THE TISSUES)

One of the early signs of kidney malfunction is excess fluid in body tissues, or a waterlogged feeling, and this is often accompanied by visible swelling around the lower limbs in particular.

Pregnancy is a time when body fluid tends to build up and cause swelling of the feet and ankles, partly because of the pressure of the growing baby on the lower abdomen, which impedes the back-flow of blood and lymph from the legs, and partly because during the middle months of pregnancy the kidneys have to filter 25 per cent more blood than before. Sometimes the contraceptive pill causes water retention, and if this happens another type of pill should be tried. Certain parts of the menstrual cycle seem to promote water retention in some women.

Whatever the cause, fluid retention must never be ignored. Minor adjustments to diet are sometimes all that is necessary to resolve the discomfort. Diuretics (pee pills) have become very popular, but taking them only makes the kidneys work harder, and though these pills may be necessary for some conditions or in the short term, it is always better to try to solve the problem at grass-roots level, i.e. by drastically cutting down on salt, especially hidden salt in processed, packaged and tinned foods. Natural diuretics such as dandelion tea can be quite effective – not for nothing did the French give it the popular name of *piss-en-lit.*

SALT

The kidneys are very involved with regulating salt levels in the blood. Nutrition expert Patrick Holford has discovered that 'saltaholics', as he calls them, can eat as much as 20g a day (more than ½oz). a day. The average person eats an estimated 12g (¼oz) a day. And the body needs a mere 3g (0.1oz) a day under normal temperatures and exertions. Salt elevates blood pressure, can cause water retention (the body's attempt to dilute salt levels) and induce stress, since it activates the fight or flight reaction of the body.

DIET FIT FOR A KIDNEY

The kidneys love water; they loathe tea and coffee. Both beverages add to their work-load, because both contain chemicals that must be excreted, as does decaffeinated coffee, which contains the chemicals needed for the decaffeination process.

Anyone with suspected kidney weakness should eat a low-protein diet, choosing protein from grains such as brown rice or lentils and not from rich red meats or shellfish. The bulk of the diet should be composed of fruit and vegetables, cooked and raw, although vegetables containing large amounts of oxalic acid, such as rhubarb and spinach, should be avoided. Avoid chocolate and cocoa. Acidic fruits, such as strawberries and tomatoes, do not always suit people with a sensitive kidney function, especially if they have a tendency to acidity – yet, that said, one of the oldest remedies for kidney stones and bladder infections is to drink the highly acidic cranberry juice.

Nature cures like with like, as all homoeopaths know, so it will not come as a surprise to learn that another excellent remedy for kidney and bladder disorders is kidney bean pod. Use 50g (2oz) fresh kidney bean pods (remove the seeds) to 4.5 litres (1 gallon) of water. Boil slowly for 4 hours, strain through a fine cloth and leave to stand for 8 hours before drinking throughout the day. Fresh supplies must be made frequently as it loses its medicinal value after 24 hours.

A combination of parsley piert and wild carrot – 25g (1oz) of each herb to 0.5 litre (1 pint) water simmered for 10 minutes then strained and refrigerated – drunk three times a day helps to clear the kidneys of deposits.

Taking magnesium has been proved to help kidney function as well. Researchers at Harvard University discovered that this mineral plus vitamin B_6 helped to prevent kidney stone formation. Prevention is always better than cure.

THE POLLUTION FACTOR

Since the kidneys must also get rid of the effects of modern pollution, especially heavy metals, it makes sense to have a hair analysis done from time to time. This is not expensive and most nutritional experts will have this done for you (see Useful Addresses, ION).

Pollution comes to us through food, water, air and, indirectly, through the tension it creates in others around us, who are, like us, striving to maintain homoeostasis in an ever-intensifying maelstrom of 20th-century life. If we can minimize just ONE part of the kidney's workload (by giving it pure water rather than tap water, which may contain unwanted substances, e.g. lead) then so much the better.

THE LYMPHATIC SYSTEM: OUR INLAND LAKE

Many people are unaware that we have two circulatory systems in the body – blood and lymph. In fact some animals have lymph hearts as well as hearts to pump blood. However we do not, and the circulation of the lymphatic fluid (a colourless or faintly opalascent fluid) is achieved by our daily muscular movements and by the process of breathing.

Lymph is the body's sap. It is a nourishing fluid, which bathes the cells and facilitates the exchange of valuable tissue foods. It also is the medium by which wastes are removed. When you have eaten poorly or drunk too much alcohol, the lymph fluid becomes clogged with wastes, and you feel waterlogged – you may even have excess fluid in certain tell-tale places, such as bags under the eyes, general facial puffiness (where there are many lymph nodes) and swollen ankles. This is because the lymph regulates fluid levels in the body, and if there are too many toxins, it simply dilutes them by increasing fluid levels.

THE LYMPH NETWORK

Besides helping the kidneys in their job of regulating fluid levels, lymph also conserves the body's protein supply, which is constantly leaking out through blood capillaries, as well as ridding the body of bacteria and other foreign particles and toxins. Its network of fluid-filled vessels is intimately connected with the blood vessel system, so that there is a constant two-way exchange.

Imagine two networks of interconnecting pipes or tunnels. By means of an elaborate system of one-way valves efferent passes from Network B (blood) to Network L (lymph). From there it is cleansed and reconditioned and then poured back into the original system. The L-system's finely-structured walls are also in touch with body cells, from which it gathers wastes formed from converting food into energy (by 'burning' it). The L-network detoxifies these by-products, filters out the wastes and returns the purified nutrients to the blood-stream. So important is this function that without it we would die of toxicosis within 24 hours.

If there is any excess fluid in body tissues it drains that out as well. Throughout the L-system network there are a series of stations or lymph nodes, in which the purification process takes place. Inside the nodes are lymph sinuses – a sinus is a place into which the body's effluent is drained – and inside those stations and their sinuses the most incredible activity takes place, because an army of small cells called lymphocytes is waiting to do its job of de-toxifying the wastes and microbes either by engulfing them or by destroying them.

Sometimes this battle between lymphocytes and microbes leads to a swelling of the lymph nodes, such as those in the neck, as more and more of them rush to combat an infection. Read more about this activity in Chapter 12.

THE LYMPHATIC SYSTEM'S VITAL PARTS

Each organ of the body has its own lymph supply. Besides these it has its own specialized network of organs. You may be surprised to read of them in the following list: spleen, thymus, tonsils and adenoids, appendix, Peyer's patches and lymph nodes . . . all are part of this complex purification system.

STAGNANT LYMPH AND ITS EFFECTS

When lymph has too much to cope with, because of a diet full of additives, preservatives, proteins and fats, it becomes sluggish and impure, like a river into which too much effluent is draining. Lymph is responsible for cholesterol conduction and for conduction of much of the fat we eat. If we eat too much fat, the lymph becomes stagnant, and in its attempts to dilute its poisons it absorbs more and more water, which then collects in the tissues, since the lymph vessels can only hold so much.

SKIN BRUSHING: MORE THAN JUST BODY POLISHING

For the average person with an occasional fluid retention and cellulite problem, one of the best ways to redress this unpleasant state of play is to improve the flow of lymph by skin brushing.

Working with dry skin (just before a bath is a good time) take a firm body brush (available from most large chemists) and, beginning with the feet, use firm strokes as if you were grooming an animal (you are!). Work up the legs back and front, up the body, sides and back, across the shoulders and up the the arms, not forgetting the surfaces like the palms of the hands and soles of the feet. Although most experts advise that you should not brush the breasts and tender parts, I don't see why they should escape – but do be gentle.

Keep at it for at least 5 minutes. After a while you will feel a wonderful tingling. This encourages elimination of toxins by the skin, assists the sloughing off of dead cells and the turnover of new ones, stimulates the lymph flow (remember this is always towards the heart so brush accordingly) and tones the entire circulation.

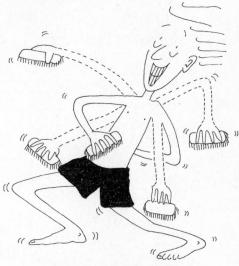

Always wash the brush after skin brushing. If you want to know why, conduct this little experiment with yourself. Brush the skin for three or four days with a damp cloth or flannel without washing it. After three or four days smell the flannel. Enough said.

Note: do not skin brush skin which is raised or abraded, such as with eczema or psoriasis. A different cleansing technique altogether must be used with these complaints – internal cleansing such as that described in Chapter 4.

You will feel a **WONDERFUL TINGLING**......

LYMPHATIC DRAINAGE MASSAGE

Most good beauty therapists perform this when they give facial massage, which is one of the reasons why one feels so marvellous afterwards. But it can be done all over. Basically it is an extremely gentle but very powerful massage treatment, which breaks down congestion in areas where lymph flow, as indicated by oedema or puffiness, has become sluggish, such as in the lower limbs or near scar tissue.

This massage can be used to advantage in treating cellulite, which is tissue in which toxic wastes have become bound into a hardened mass. It not only stimulates the eliminatory functions of the lymphatic system but also helps to stimulate the immune system by encouraging the proliferation of lymphocytes.

AROMATHERAPY: MILLION-DOLLAR MASSAGE

Many women say they feel better after they have been to the beauty parlour or had their hair styled. Those same women would feel heaps better still if they budgeted for a weekly aromatherapy session.

Quite apart from the fact that the massage concentrates on lymphatic drainage, it also applies itself to the nervous system, thus relieving tension in the spine. The use of essential oils to heighten the effect simply adds to the magic of the treatment, for all the senses are bathed in soothing experiences, the ears with the soft music that is played, the skin with the sensation of touch, and the nose with the wonderful natural aromas of the oils, while the eyes are rested under pads of soothing eye lotion.

The technique actually releases the aromatic hydrocarbons in the oils into the lymphatic system where they cleanse, tone and stimulate the antimicrobial action of lymph. The type of oil is chosen to suit the client's condition. Commonly used oils are those such as lemon or bergamot; others include juniper, pennyroyal or patchouli, which are used to combat oedema; yet others such as sandalwood, thyme, rosemary and cinnamon are used to aid in the purification of the lymph itself.

Benefits continue after the treatment is over, and I have often thought it is a pity that men do not avail themselves of aromatherapy more. It has a beauty parlour connotation that unfortunately excludes it from the very sex who may need it most.

THE DIET: LYMPH ENLIVENER

Here is a cleansing diet aimed at de-clogging the lymphatic system in order to encourage it to eliminate its wastes more easily.

Eat only apples or grapes for a week end. (Use one variety only.) During the following week or so eliminate all dairy foods, such as cheese, butter, cream and milk, all red meats, vinegar, alcohol, refined carbohydrates and all processed canned and packaged food, plus artificial colourings, preservatives and salty foods and sweets, chocolates, ice cream . . . the works.

Be prepared to get a headache; this is caused by your grateful body being able to eliminate stored toxins. Then take a course of echinacea drops or tablets (called prairie doctor in the US). This neutralizes acidity and promotes the production of lymphocytes.

THE SKIN

The skin actually forms a vital part of another body system called the integumentary system, consisting of the skin, hair and nails, all of which are composed of variations of roughly the same substances. They are designed to protect the body from foreign invaders and from wear and tear, and they are part of our external armoury. However, the eliminatory functions of the skin are so vital and so often overlooked, that I have elected to position them in this chapter in order to emphasize this aspect as being one which we should promote. I believe it can bring better help to the kidneys in their herculean task of coping with our toxicity-laden 20th-century bodies!

There is an added bonus to encouraging this function; the techniques recommended, such as skin brushing, will help to keep skin supple and beautiful. And the dietary measures suggested will help to dispel cellulite, that plague of our current dietary habits.

SKIN STRUCTURE

About 19,350 sq cm (3,000 sq in) of skin cover our bodies. It is the largest organ we possess and amounts of 15 per cent of our body weight. One square inch of skin has about 250 sweat glands, 25 hairs, 40 sebaceous glands, 2.3m (7ft 6in) of blood vessels, 11m (30ft) of nerves and 7,500 sensory cells. Wow! Another one of the body's compact miracles.

Unlike any other organ of the body, the skin is directly and continuously exposed to the environment, acting as our protective mantle to ward off heat and cold, bacteria, dust, pollutants and the slings and arrows of life. It also has the vital function of keeping water in and keeping water out, plus all the characteristics mentioned earlier. Together with its sister tissues, hair and nails, it is the best reflector of health we have, as well as being a pretty fair indicator of psychological states. It surely is the only organ we have that can go red, pink, blue, yellow, white, brown, purple or ashen, and that is quite apart from unwelcome decorations that render it spotty, blotchy, pimply, scaly, wrinkled, furrowed or pockmarked.

It is the prime organ of touch as well, under the influence of which it can tingle, flush, bristle, shrink, or glow. It semaphores our emotions to the world and also, through itching, weeping and bleeding, our suffering.

It manufactures vitamin D, controls body temperature, provides sexual attraction and signals racial origin.

And it is unique. Our skin patterns are shared by no one. This is particularly true of the palms of our hands and the soles of our feet, around which a whole study, Chirology, has been formulated, but equally is it unique in parts that seldom get scrutinized.

Skin is composed of different layers, each layer having its own properties. In this sense it resembles plywood, and as such is much stronger than a single layer of corresponding thickness.

177

There are two chief layers, the dermis, or underlayer, and the epidermis or surface layer. Beneath them there is a layer of fat, our padding. In reality the epidermis consists of several layers of cells, which are constantly rising to the surface and being replaced by the wear and tear of life. These cells, especially those nearest to the surface, are for the most part dead, but they are extremely orderly in their arrangement and they do contain water, which is essential for the skin's suppleness and flexibility.

There are no blood cells in the outer epidermis, but there are melanocytes, and these produce the pigment melanin, which protects us against the sun and is responsible for tanning. It is also responsible for the colour of darker skinned people; oddly enough the blondest

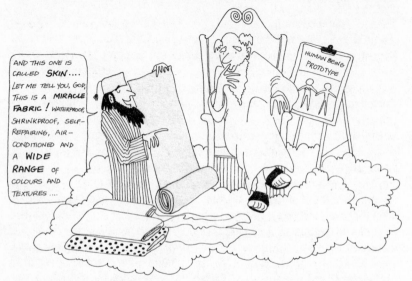

Scandinavian has as many melanocytes as the darkest negro – however they do not have the facility to produce melanin in the quantity and quality of those from countries exposed to hot sun.

The deepest part of the epidermis is the zone of germination, where the still-living cells are constantly dividing and moving slowly to the surface. It takes about 28 days for a cell to rise from this deepest layer to the surface, which is about as long as a suntan lasts if you don't peel!

In a lifetime we shed no fewer than 18kg (40lb) of skin because of this constant replacement programme. As the cells rise to the surface they steadily acquire a filling of keratin, which hardens them and makes them more protective. Most people have heard of keratin in respect of hair, and it is true that both hair and nails are composed of this same substance, although it is arranged in different densities.

The dermis is, if anything, even more complex than the epidermis, and it is from this generative layer that all major skin glands arise, as well as hair follicles. The dermis is a dense layer of cells, which are full of the protein collagen, and these, together with elastic fibres, give skin its pliability and strength.

Here lies a rich supply of blood vessels, far more than the skin needs for its own nutrition. This gives the clue to one of its most important functions other then elimination: heat control. An ingenious system of shunts between the outgoing arterial and returning venous blood supply enable blood to be directed to the tiny capillaries which traverse the skin if heat loss is desired, or completely bypass it if heat conservation is required. This is no doubt why we look pinker in warm weather and pinched and white in the cold.

To a certain extent this tremendous flexibility allows control of blood pressure as well.

Another cooling measure is supplied by sweat glands. When it is hot, these glands pour water onto the skin's surface, where evaporation cools it. Some of the sweat glands, the apocrines, are responsible for our characteristic body smell, which is a throwback to our hairier ancestors, who clearly had to attract each other from the trees!

Interspersed among the sweat glands are the sebaceous glands, which secrete an oily substance that lubricates both skin and hair. These are attached to hair follicles, and they pour their secretions onto the hair as it grows. It is an interesting fact that this production is linked to the production of androgen, a male hormone. Both men and women produce each other's hormones to some degree, and it is minute amounts of androgen that give women their 'get-up-and-go'. Presumably our oilier and possibly hairier brothers and sisters have higher androgen levels.

One other group of cells and their network are well in evidence in the skin, and that is the lymphatic system, making lymph drainage a vital factor in skin function. As a first line of protection, the skin plays a major role in immune function, and it is as well to know that anything on the skin – a patch or fixed dressing, for example – interferes with lymph drainage in that area.

NUTRITION AND THE SKIN

There is a great deal of controversy as to whether facial creams and lotions do actually penetrate the skin and have nutritional value. As vitamins are given this way to people too ill to digest them and oestrogen is absorbed this way from the patches of hormone replacement therapy, it seems likely that some benefit is derived.

However, the chief source of nutrition for the skin comes from within and seeps up from the dermis through the fluid-filled spaces between the cells. In the epidermis these cells are joined together with zipper-like contacts, so it is easy for fluids to penetrate between the contacts.

The skin needs all the vitamins but its particular affinity is with vitamin A. This is best taken in the form of pro-vitamin A or beta-carotene (found in carrots and yellow vegetables and fruits), as this form of vitamin A cannot become toxic in high doses as can retinol.

Liposomes and humectants (substances that moisturize and give body to the skin) are also vital and should always be supplied in good skin preparations. When on holiday a simple aerosol containing the skin's own natural moisturizer, NaCPA, should be sprayed on the skin. It is available from good health product suppliers such as Nature's Best in the UK (see Useful Addresses). The same company also supplies natural beta-carotene.

AIDING ELIMINATION: GENERAL AND SPECIFIC (CELLULITE).
If you have patches of skin resembling the skin of an orange, the odds are that you have dieted too quickly at some stage and that you may have eaten the wrong foods. The important thing is not to castigate yourself for not knowing what you know now (or will know in a minute) and not to give up, but to accept that what took quite a lot of unknowing effort to achieve will take an equal amount of knowing effort to undo!

The effects will be dazzling. You will look and feel so much better that you may even cease to worry whether the cellulite is there or not!

There is no single cause to cellulite or a single effective treatment; only an overall plan of detoxification, exercise and massage will do the trick. Cellulite starts with the predisposition of all women to have a goodly layer of fat under their skin. This is a by-product of the female hormone oestrogen, which is why men rarely suffer from the affliction. It is also why cellulite usually starts when the hormone levels are being tinkered with in some way, either through natural processes such as puberty or pregnancy, or by the less natural ones of going on the pill.

There is usually the complication of a tendency to retain fluid, which is often caused by sluggish lymph. To keep lymph flowing plenty of movement is needed; sedentary lifestyles positively promote cellulite. However, it is as true to say that professional women athletes suffer from it. The situation is a complex one. Basically, the fluids that have escaped from the tissues get bound up with fat and the wastes it contains (fat is inert and the body uses it to store toxins it has not been able to eliminate). In a sense, cellulite is a protective substance, a kind of nuclear waste disposal section. The fact that is is so hard to re-absorb tells how successful is this little body venture.

Most women with cellulite try all kinds of expensive and painful therapies such as liposuction, lymph drainage, and ionithermie, but these do not get to the bottom (thigh, hip, upper arm!) of the problem. The only thing that will is a general de-toxification and elimination programme, measures such as are described in the diet and herbs lymph enlivener (see above), combined with a complete review of general diet (see Chapter 4). Skin-brushing also helps.

One of the commonest skin conditions is acne, and it causes terrible suffering, partly because it happens to adolescents right at the time when they want to look their best. Its onset in puberty is occasioned by the increase in hormone production, in particular androgens, which are produced in girls by their adrenal glands and in boys by both the testes and adrenals. This hormone has an effect on the sebaceous glands, prompting them to produce more oil. This can block pores, which in turn can become infected, which causes the pimple to form.

Treatment is best done by natural means and not by taking a lengthy course of antibiotics, which will interfere with the intestinal flora, setting the adolescent up for more trouble later. If a course of antibiotics is deemed necessary, bio-yoghurt should always be taken at the same time.

Washing the face in mild soap – castile or ivory, for example – and water two or three times a day helps, as does eliminating commercial shampoos for shampooing the hair. Eliminate all oily and fatty foods from the diet, which should be composed of raw food, fresh fruits and vegetables. Take only 1 tablespoon of cold-pressed soybean, sesame or flaxseed oil, preferably a salad dressing, daily.

Healthy diets are hard for some adolescents to follow, yet they respond so quickly to them. It may also help to take plenty of pro-vitamin A in beta-carotene form (get nutritional advice on the quantity), as well as plenty of niacin (vitamin B_3), which brings blood to the surface of the skin and so improves drainage. Use only non-allergenic cosmetics or facial preparations and buy small sizes, which will be replaced frequently and so have less tendency to get infected. Always wash hands before applying.

Other more serious skin complaints are not the domain of a general guide book such as this. However, it should be said that the single factor of a good diet will do much to alleviate most of them, because such a diet (see Chapter 4) will support the elimination and immune functions of the body, allowing nature to cure the skin condition.

11

*

THE IMMUNE SYSTEM

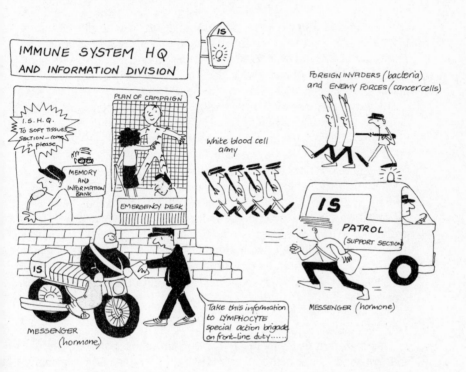

IN THIS CHAPTER

* The whiter-than-white immune army * Antibody
activity * The thymus and its T-cells * The meaning of
auto-immune * Testing your unwellness level * For 'allergy'
read 'early warning'; for 'help' read 'homoeopathy' * The
seven enemies of health * How our illnesses reflect our
conflicts * Killer diseases and how to conquer them
* Boosting your immune system

Time was when virtually nobody knew what an immune system was, and that time was not very long ago – pre-AIDS, in fact. Now it has the highest profile of any system in the body – yet where is it?

The immune system is quite literally everywhere. Omnipresent in the body, like a benign police force, it patrols the blood, bone and soft tissues, on constant alert for anything that threatens the body's well-being.

Most people have heard of white blood cells, which are given the general name of leucocytes. This army of tiny, one-celled organisms together with the action-prompting 'messenger' hormones released and which they in turn release, control and orchestrate the immune response killing invaders such as bacteria and viruses, and destroying unhealthy body cells. For their efforts white blood cells live very short lives – only about 10 days, while red blood cells live for 120 days. The life of a soldier has always been short and hard.

However, they are very resourceful. Unlike red blood cells, which simply get swept along in the bloodstream, white blood cells can move of their own volition, which is how they can get to the site of an infection. They can even move through the walls of normally impermeable blood vessels in order to protect whatever surrounding tissue seems to need them. Fortunately, they are made, at the rate of 2,000 a second if you are in good health, in different sites of the body so that if one area becomes deactivated or undermined, other parts will take over their production. The chief sites of production are primarily the bone marrow and secondarily the liver, lymph glands and spleen. The thymus gland, which is part of the endocrine system, is also involved in white cell production, in this case in perfecting one group of them called T-cells (see below).

THE WHITE CELL BRIGADE

Just as there are divisions in the army, each with its special purpose, so there are divisions in the white cell brigade. Yet originally and initially, a bit like clones, they all arise from the same stem cell, which is produced in the bone marrow. Some of these stem cells will become red blood corpuscles, some platelets, which are responsible for blood clotting, and the rest will become any one of several different kinds of white blood cells, all of which are concerned with attacking foreign invaders, including tissue that the body itself throws up from time to time which they are not happy with such as cancer cells. The body is not perfect: it has its production line faults and rejects, very often produced under the stress of too many working hours, too little sleep and so on.

The stem cells which transform into white blood cells form four main divisions of the immune system. One group, the B-lymphocytes, is concerned with repelling foreign invaders such as bacteria and a few viruses;

the other, the T-lymphocytes (of which there are four sub-divisions), is concerned more with the recognition and rejection of foreign tissue, such as the above-mentioned cancer cells, or any foreign particle, such as a fungus, which gets into the bloodstream. It is these cells which prompt the rejection of skin or organ transplants from other donors; regrettably you cannot tell them just this once not to do their job.

The other two divisions constitute the firing line and support sections for the front-line attackers. These are the granulocytes (called neutrophils, basophils and eosiniphils) and the monocytes. The granulocytes, and in particular the neutrophils, are the first on the scene when a foreign invader such as a stomach 'bug' bacteria strikes. They are lucky if they live 6 hours and 100 billion of them get wiped out each day – more during a nasty infection, which means a similar number of replacements have to be made. Once the neutrophils have found their target, they ingest it. In so doing they are helped by certain enzymes which are released and which actually make the bacteria more tasty. But bacteria are 'junk food' after all, and their ingestion hastens the death of the neutrophils.

Then the second line of defence, the monocytes, takes over, and these help to clean up the battlefield of all the dead bodies. They also stimulate the production of more neutrophils. They are involved in the immune system's chemical warfare, which is designed to deactivate, by one means or another, the body's microbial, toxic and self-generated enemies.

ANTIBODY ACTIVITY

Two very powerful divisions of the immune system, the B-lymphocytes and the T-lymphocytes, have the job of remembering the body's past invaders and forming small groups of memory cells that will recognize this particular invader in future. Thus it is that a first attack of measles will be very severe, and the person will feel ill while the war wages between the measles germs and the immune system. But if the germs try to invade a second time, the system will not be caught unprepared: it will immediately know how to deal with this particular invader, and its host will suffer few, if any, symptoms.

The T-cells work in a similar way to the B-cells, but instead of producing antibodies they produce substances called lymphokines, which are the immune system's natural drugs. An example of these substances are interferons, well-known for their demonstrated ability to fight cancer and inhibit virus multiplication and cell division. The substances produced by the T-lymphocytes are frequently involved in many allergic reactions, particularly the delayed ones such as the headache or migraine that occur some hours after ingesting a food to which there is an allergy. Food allergies are becoming more and more common because we are eating food that is not natural and very often full of toxic chemicals for preservation purposes as well. All cooked and processed food is recognized by the immune system as a threat, a foreign invader, so the simple act of eating cooked food actually activates our immune system responses. (Always eat something raw before each meal.)

THE MEANING OF AUTO-IMMUNE DISEASES

Like all armies, unless they are properly maintained and stringently controlled, the divisions of the immune system can become disorderly. A poorly functioning immune system ceases to know the difference between the enemy and host, and when this happens it attacks its own cells, which is what happens in the case of auto-immune diseases such as rheumatoid arthritis, ankylosing spondylitis, motor neurone disease, systemic lupus, myasthenia gravis, pernicious anaemia and even some kinds of diabetes. In these cases, distorted cell chemistry and activity actually affect the cells' behaviour, just as alcohol affects the brain when imbibed in too great quantities, the difference being that in the former case the effects are there all the time; in the latter, the imbiber will sober up!

The only way out of this maze is to embark on a complete body-cleanse during which the toxins etc. that are befuddling the immune system are eliminated (see Gerson Cancer Therapy, Useful Addresses).

During antibody activity histamine is produced, and sometimes this reaction is excessive, producing all the classic signs of allergy, such as asthma, hay fever or urticaria. These frightening and seemingly wanton acts of the body are simply signs that a highly sophisticated system is malfunctioning due to dietary or lifestyle overload or omissions. Vitamin C is a natural antihistamine, which is why it is so wise to take extra vitamin C (2–3g) if you suffer from hay fever or any infection that alerts the immune system.

THE THYMUS AND T-CELLS

The thymus gland, which is situated under the main central 'bump' of the breastbone, used to be considered redundant by the time we reached teenage. Now it is known that it is a chief organizer of the immune response, issuing instructions via a group of hormones, of which thymosin is one, which act as runners or messengers to the body's defence systems.

So vital is the role of the thymus and its production of the four sub-groups of T-lymphocytes, that the deficiency of any one group of them can lead to serious impairment of immune function.

This is what happens with AIDS, in which the virus HTLV III or HIV destroys the T-helper cells, leaving the sufferer inadequately defended against certain infections and in particular against the incidence of cancer. On the other hand, a deficiency in T-suppressor cells, which regulate and control excessive immune responses, results in autoimmune diseases. Here the immune system behaves like an army on the rampage, marauding and killing willy-nilly.

Thus a deficiency in any one of the sub-divisions can be seen to render the body vulnerable to one set of diseases or another. The solution lies in repairing damaged immune function, not in treating the result of that dysfunction – the disease. The fact that this may entail a lengthy programme of slow but sure rehabilitation is becoming increasingly accepted in our new understanding of 21st-century health – the real aim of which is prevention.

THE UNWELL TEST: WHEN DOES UNEASE BECOME DISEASE?

Illness does not happen overnight; it is the sum total of many days and nights of ignoring early symptoms of unease, precursor of the more serious state that comes later – disease. Again, the richness of our language gives the clue we tend to ignore: the difference between unease and disease is just a question of degree. Or, put another way, wellness ... unwellness ... illness! So take stock when you feel unwell, don't wait until illness strikes. Review the lifestyle and diet (including emotional diet) that may be contributing to this deterioration. Make it part of your daily routine to examine yourself.

Take stock of your dreams – what are they telling you? Start with a morning routine, which involves the physical; then in the evening recap on the day and see how you feel on the psychological plane.

Where and how do you start? What about in the bathroom mirror when you get up in the morning!

UNEASE PROFILE: PASSING YOUR "PHYSICAL"
Eyes are the windows of the soul, they say. They are also the mirrors of the body – in fact iris diagnosis (diagnosis of physical conditions from a close examination of the eyes) is based on known correspondences between parts of the eye and parts of the body. And very accurate it is, too. So start with your eyes as prime indicators of health. Observe these daily, and also any changes in nails, hair, and colour of skin. This is the physical appearance we should check in the morning – not the vanity one!

Check if you have any of the following unease details and score minus one for each. Start with a score of 30.

● Eyes: yellowed whites, bloodshot, gravelly, watery, pain on movement, dark circles or bags underneath.

● Hair: dry/greasy, dandruff, colour/texture deterioration, lowered growth rate.

● Nails: ridged vertically or horizontally, brittle, white or blue, hourglass, flecks, split.

● Colour of skin on face and palms of hands: yellowish, greyish, transparent, blotchy.

● Ears: noises, bubbles, itchy, noises far away, own voice loud.

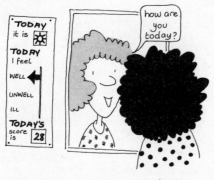

MAKE IT PART OF YOUR DAILY ROUTINE TO EXAMINE YOURSELF.....

● Nose: runny, itchy, sore, difficulty in breathing, loss of smell.

● Mouth: bad taste, bad breath, coated tongue, ulcers, loss of taste, bleeding gums.

● Body skin: spots, rashes, colour change, dry/flaky, tight, change in number or appearance of moles, body odour.

● Throat: itchy, sore, swollen glands, difficulty swallowing.

● Head: tight, dull ache, woozy, dizzy, pain on movement.

● Joints: stiff, weak, swollen, painful.

Deduct more than seven? Still convinced your health is OK? Deduct on through the following symptoms:

● Digestion: heartburn, flatulence, bloating, persistent constipation or diarrhoea.

● Sleep: altered patterns, worrying dreams.

● Energy levels: very affected by what you eat, drink, are told (good news/bad news).

● Appetite and weight: unsatisfactory changes.

● Sex drive: lowered or sporadic.

● Allergies and food sensitivities: increasing?

● Menstrual cycle: worsening PMT or other changes.

188

● Hyperactivity (unable to switch off and rest when you do have the chance).

● Changes in handwriting.

Deduct more than five here? Still convinced your health is A1? Now deduct a point for answering each and any of the following questions in the affirmative:

● Have you been avoiding social gatherings lately because they make you tired?

● Do you lack sufficient exercise of a kind that gets the heart beating fast at least 20 minutes a day? Or do you lack the time or impetus to take a half hour's brisk daily walk?

● Are you unhappy with a major aspect of your life?

● Do you often/regularly take drugs/medicines?

● Are you hopeless without cigarettes, coffee, strong tea or alcohol during the day?

● Do you heal slowly?

● Do you get easily upset, angry, anxious or irritable?

● Do you eat a lot of refined or convenience foods such as sandwiches?

● Do you rarely eat raw fruit or vegetables?

● Have you had any major life changes lately?

Five deductions or more should be making you think a lot.

Remember: illness doesn't happen overnight. It sometimes takes two, three, four or even five decades for an illness to develop, an illness you were probably warned about by your immune system in childhood.

ALLERGY: THE VERY EARLY WARNING SIGN
An allergy can be defined as an abnormally heightened sensitivity to a substance (allergen) on the part of the immune system.

Allergies usually start in childhood when, like childhood diseases, they are rarely taken seriously. But childhood diseases and conditions – both your own and those of your child – should never be viewed as a natural part of growing up. A health history should be taken and attempts made to eradicate from the system the miasmas or overloads or effects of such illnesses. This is best done in childhood, where the body is new, young and strong; it can also be done in adulthood but with more difficulty.

Allergy is one of the earliest signs of stress in the body. There is not just one type of allergy – a reaction to pollen or house dust – there are environmental and food allergies as well. Some people actually inherit a tendency to be allergic. Whatever the cause or provocation, allergies are warning signs. They are the first yellow or cautionary flags of the immune system. If they are not addressed the body simply learns to live with them, suppressing the acute symptoms for most of the time so that you can get on with your life. But the first little snake has claimed its victim in the snakes and ladders of life.

Today we have an alarming picture of the incidence of childhood allergies increasing by, some say, as much as 30 per cent. Yet it is not believed that this is allergy in the classic sense – that is, an excessive response by the immune system to the typical allergens of house dust, grass and tree pollen, shellfish, strawberries, animal fur and so on. Only 1 per cent of the population traditionally suffers from this kind of allergic reaction.

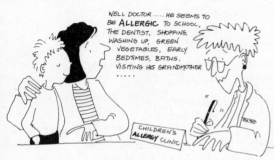

What are the other 29 per cent suffering from? People like Dr Jean Monro, a UK specialist in the treatment of allergies, (who, together with Dr Peter Mansfield, has written a chilling book on children and allergy, *Chemical Children*) believes that we are witnessing an allergic reaction to what in broadest terms could be called the 20th century. In effect this suggests that current environmental factors and pressures are weakening the defences of all of us – that is, we are suffering a system overload rather than a simple allergy. The fact that our children are suffering the most is because, in Dr Monro's opinion, it is always the newer generation that is badly affected.

The following symptoms may all be signs of allergic reactions: nausea, digestive upsets (especially bloating), breathing difficulties and constricted throat, headaches, chronic catarrh, skin rashes or weals, mouth ulcers, menstrual disorders, nervous/mental conditions such as disturbing or agressive behaviour, aching joints, lack of muscular co-ordination or hyperactivity.

There are three main groups of culprits responsible for this alarming rise in the body's yellow flags of caution: 20th-century diet, 20th-century environmental pollution and 20th-century lifestyles. They are all contributing in different measures to what might be called 'incipient toxicology'.

Allergies and their causes are so difficult to pin down that it is understandable when a busy family doctor glosses over them, or prescribes antihistamine tablets, which suppress the unpleasant symptoms but do not attack the underlying problem.

It is up to the sufferer to make a dossier, noting every possible action or food eaten that preceded a bad attack. Environmental factors should not be discounted, including local trees and grasses, living near a main road, the presence of polluted water (including household water supplies), sprays used by the council, household chemicals used in cleaning or pesticides used in the garden. Local factories or activities with chemicals that require powerful sources of electricity should also be considered, as well as personal clothing, cosmetics and creams, perfumes, bed linen, house dust, toys and so on – the list is very long but every individual has a very strong ally in their sixth sense.

TREATMENT OPTIONS

Homoeopathy addresses allergies better than orthodox medicine because it begins with the basic premise 'one sick patient is to be studied, not the disease'. It is known that allergies can strike just one person in a large family, all of whom are living the same lifestyle and eating the same diet. Or it may affect two members in different ways.

One of the distinguishing characteristics of homoeopathy is that it maintains that a patient's susceptibility to infections, whether bacterial, fungal or viral, is preceded by organic susceptibility. In other words, there has to be an innate weakness there in the first place – the allergen merely brings it out.

Every single person has a weakness of some kind in one system of the body or another. Weaknesses in the immune system give rise to such widespread symptoms of such variety because the immune system is omnipresent. They are the hardest to track down, because of this and because the severity of the symptoms varies – one day the immune system may be functioning better than another because the diet was more sensible on that day, or the person slept better, or a happy event occurred in the family.

The homoeopathic approach should always be chosen in the instance of conditions that come and go such as allergies. Diet must be reviewed and as many factors as possible removed from the diet which could be adding to the strain, such as food containing additives.

Parents who have a child suffering from an allergy should try any or all of the following:

1. Change all household products and all washing powders to bio-degradable.

2. Change a great portion of the diet to fresh and organic produce.
3. Give the child bottled water, preferably from glass containers.
4. Try to eliminate as many synthetic and dust-catching agents as possible – some soft toys may have to go.
5. Try to vary the diet so that the same food is not eaten every day.
6. See that some exercise is taken in less polluted areas.
7. Do not allow the ingestion of too much fat, from chips, for example, because it clogs the immune systems.

When an allergy has been present for some time, the sufferer needs to have a rest from the allergen so that the system can quieten down. Sometimes the offending substance is then re-introduced to see just how severe the reaction is.

Some allergic conditions are akin to alcoholism in that the person actually craves the thing that is bad for them, and when this happens it takes time for the conditioned response to return to normal. When it does there will be a violent reaction to the previously craved substance.

ARE YOU SLEEPING IN A HEALTHY PLACE?

Environmental 'allergies' are becoming more and more prevalent and can be extremely subtle in their effects. Some interesting studies have been done in families where there are several children, one of whom is poorly, sleeping in the same room. Dowsers have found that certain earth rays that pass through walls may be concentrated in the place where the ill child is sleeping. In these days of increasing electromagnetic pollution from household sources such as television and computers, as well as from the outside environment, it is well worth the small expense of having the household area dowsed if a family member is inexplicably unwell (see Useful Addresses). Sometimes all that is needed is a simple re-positioning of a bed or domestic electrical equipment. Dowsers usually work under a group or association, and these can be found by looking in health directories or inquiring from health editors or publications devoted to this kind of interest.

HOUSE DUST AND HOUSE MITES

This is one of the commonest causes of allergic reactions within the home and the simple formula given here can be made up by your local pharmacist and sprayed about the house. It has a mite-terminating effect and smells very pleasant: 2 parts oil of juniper, 10 parts naptha, 5 parts camphor, 10 parts phenic acid, 5 parts lemon oil, 2 parts thyme oil, 2 parts lavender oil; all to be mixed in 500 parts of rectified spirits.

THE ENEMIES OF HEALTH AND THE IMMUNE SYSTEM

Dr Alfred Vogel, a pioneer in the New Health Movement, lists the following as the arch-eroders of good health, producing allergic reactions as well as diseases that undermine future health.

1. Fungi
2. Bacteria
3. Viruses
4. Parasites
5. Diseases caused by deficencies and allergies
6. Overeating
7. Poisons

Apropos this list, here is the current situation. In the last 10 to 20 years we have seen an alarming increase in the severity of the effects of certain viruses and fungi on general health, such as Coxsackie, varicella zoster and Epstein-Barr viruses, which can feature in ME and *Candida albicans*, the yeast-like organism that can become, under certain conditions, fungal in nature, penetrate the wall of the gut and thereafter pour toxins into the bloodstream.

These, together with the increasing incidence of allergies, PMT and infections like ME, resistant strains of VD, infectious hepatitis and AIDS, are challenging health authorities and their resources to the extreme. And never forget that many of the drugs we are given, which are further polluting our insides, are the very chemicals that have been prescribed for us in order to fight the conditions described above!

Are germs getting stronger or are we getting weaker?

What seems to be happening is the kind of situation that occurred in *Gulliver's Travels*, when the Lilliputians slowly but surely rendered the 'giant' totally defenceless. The Lilliputian cocktail is deadly, and it consists of many interlinking threads, including polluting agents in the air, water and earth, chemicals used in industry and introduced into foods either while they are being grown or while they are being processed, the chemicals we use in household and garden products and so forth. Even the ingestion today of what might on the surface seem like a wholesome meal of meat and three (fresh) vegetables, unless each has been organically grown, can contain hormones, pesticides and other residues, to say nothing of the eroding effects on remaining nutritional values occasioned by modern cooking processes.

THE FOOD 'FAMINE'

Immune cells need nutrients. Much of the food we eat today is lacking in certain vital trace minerals such as selenium and zinc. Zinc is probably the mineral most lacking in British diets, yet it is vital to certain body processes. A more detailed profile of today's nutritional food plight is given in Chapter 4, but it needs to be included in the discussion of immune function.

This is not scaremongering. Big business, right up to government level, is turning towards profits and away from the modern research that indicates all too clearly how public health is being eroded by pollution, faulty nutrition and very often by prescribed drugs that do little more than pour oil on the troubled waters of health conditions (and money into the coffers of drug companies).

What can the ordinary person do? A great deal. We may not be able to change big business, which has always been profit orientated, but we can change our lifestyles and we can take control of what goes into our bodies. We can create a demand for food that is wholesome, for products that are safe and for medicines that are natural, and in doing so we will force their price down as surely as the Lilliputians brought down Gulliver. The alternative is domination by an outdated health system.

IMMUNE SYSTEM UNDERMINERS

Bearing the above in mind, experts agree that the following factors also feature:

1. Removal of tonsils
2. Diet high in refined carbohydrates, low in complex carbohydrates and low in trace minerals.
3. Previous illnesses involving the liver, pancreas, spleen, kidneys and lymph system.
4. Social drugs, including marijuana.
5. Many sexual partners.
6. Emotional or mental stressors, including those that inspire feelings of guilt, shame, rejection and failure.
7. Inability to express anger (and other strong emotions).

Points 6 and 7 highlight the significance of mental and emotional conditions, which are now known to have an effect on immune system functioning. What has been known intrinsically for many hundreds of years – that people do get sick after a death in the family or a serious life change – has now been proved by the new science of psychneuroimmunology. This mouthful of word simply means there is a brand new science to study the pathways whereby unhappiness gets into our cells (see Chapter 7).

HOW OUR ILLNESSES REFLECT OUR CONFLICTS

The type of experiences life brings to us and how we handle them are reflected in the illnesses we may develop. For example, as long ago as Solomon's day the classic rheumatoid arthritic personality was described as follows: she is likely to be more of a masochist or long-suffering female, denying any feelings of hostility to those she serves with compliance, reacting with great sensitivity to shows of anger, and with a history of being nervous, tense, worried, highly-strung and moody. If it were not so sad, it would be fascinating to observe how well the body expresses this character profile in the auto-immune disease of rheumatoid arthritis, in which the immune system attacks its own body cells.

There are personality profiles to go with all the major killer diseases. Cardio-vascular people are usually high achievers; cancer sufferers have become negative about something. Of course, there are physical and environmental factors too.

Does this mean our diseases are inevitable? Not at all. Such awareness should serve only to warn us that that we cannot leave our health entirely to our doctors: we must keep a constant vigilance on both our innate vulnerabilities and our current pressures. Even so, serious disease can surprise us – although it is never too late to restore health.

THE ADVENT OF SERIOUS DISEASE

Those people puffing away on cigarettes or eating rich diets do not really believe that they will ever get cancer or arterial disease. In youth and middle age it is so easy to believe that those life-threatening diseases happen to other people. Most people get a terrible shock when they are given the bad news that they have a serious illness, and the shock itself further depletes the immune system. Then they rally – the 'this can't happen to me' feeling is born. This is the first sign of the fighter coming into being, and it is good.

But then they go for treatment and the treatment (a) further upsets them by reminding them that they are ill and (b) very often makes them feel worse. But they have been told, as a kind of sentence, that that is the treatment they must go through in order to get better.

Wrong. There are always choices; there are always alternatives. So before further stressing your immune system by beginning treatment that consists of drugs, which may further poison and undermine what is already serious, consider the alternatives. Go to see experts who practise them. Consider carefully before starting any treatment. A week or two of intensive investigation, reading and consultations about your illness will not hasten your demise, but it will enable you to make informed decisions about **your** body.

Those with arterial disease should read the chapter on circulation, particularly the alternative to orthodox treatment, chelation. Those suffering from cancer, whatever decisions they make, should consider radical changes in their diets, such as is advocated by some highly successful alternative therapies such as the Gerson Cancer Therapy. There are others, but this one is briefly described here because of the meticulous case histories have kept for a very long time pertaining to many different kinds of cancer. (Read *Cancer Therapy: Results of 50 Cases* by Dr Max Gerson – see Useful Addresses.)

Treatment is based on a vegetarian diet and the ingestion, hourly at first, of fresh organic vegetable and fruit juices to restore cellular health. It uses coffee enemas to speed up the excretion of toxins that have accumulated in the tissues. Although this diet has become known as the Gerson cancer therapy, it was never specifically designed for cancer, and it works as well with any serious disease, including AIDS. It does require dedication and total abandonment of all the practices that have led up to the illness in the first place, which, regrettably, few sufferers are prepared to do.

It is based on the principle that a healthy immune system will deal with disease, even serious disease, when given the right support. But first the toxins which have accumulated in the cells and which are responsible for the distortion of immune system function, have to be eradicated, by a diet of fresh, living food in the intensely compact form of fruit and vegetable juices.

For this reason all fruits and vegetables used in Gerson therapy must be organically grown. Essentially the therapy consists of two major processes, the detoxifying one and the rebuilding and purifying one. And it is all done with diet!

If ever we needed to know what a powerful tool for health (or sickness) diet is, this therapy, which has been seen to work for people at death's door, should prove it to us. However, one thing is known: it is much more difficult to cure people who have been treated with chemotherapy than those who have not.

There is now a school of thought that believes that cancer viruses, bacteria and fungi may be the same basic organism at different stages of their cycle. All the more reason to take fungal and viral infections seriously, before they become their more serious relative. (Those interested in knowing more about this line of thought should read about the work of Gaston Naessens – see Useful Addresses).

GET WELL THERAPIES

Apart from diet and positive visualization, in which the person visualizes their immune system fighting the disease – a form of biofeedback (see Chapter 7), acupuncture has proved successful in that it prompts the release of the body's natural hormones, endorphins, which in turn prompt the production of more T-cells. Acupressure or Shiatsu work equally well in some cases, the latter being particularly effective with AIDS, as are most of the therapies involving therapeutic touch and massage. Touch therapies are all-important in serious illness, yet people who are very ill often feel unloved and unclean – untouchable – so that others shun them. We are all afraid of illness, and we turn away instead of turning towards, forgetting it might be us next time.

Gerson therapy can be learned and practised in the home. Other therapies that seem to help and that have been mentioned in various chapters in this book include: anthroposophical medicine, which examines every aspect of a patient's life (see Chapter 12); the self-help technique of meditation (active visualization) which has also proved helpful in organizing and marshalling the immune system defences, as have certain herbal substances and adaptogens, especially Shitake and Reishi mushrooms (see Chapter 4). Lapacho and echinacea have also helped with degenerative diseases. Let a naturopath or herbalist advise you.

People with heart conditions need to recognize their self-achievement pattern and learn to relax, to switch off. Biofeedback techniques, forms of meditation or walking several miles a day, preferably in green surroundings, will help to restore both circulation and balance.

RECIPE FOR A SOUND IMMUNE SYSTEM

I took this recipe from the excellent booklet *How to Boost Your Immune System* written by Jennifer Meek and published by ION (see Useful Addresses).

'Assuming you are not on any special diet for medical reasons, these basic guidelines will serve you daily for the rest of your life.

● Of the total calorific intake, 60% should be taken in carbohydrate form comprising grains other than exclusively wheat (our national addiction) and lots of fresh fruit and vegetables.

● Not more than 20% should come from fat, making sure that this contains the essential fatty acids, especially linoleic acid (e.g. sunflower and safflower oils) and EPA (seafood and cod liver oil).

● The remaining 20% should come from protein (ensuring all the amino acids, if vegetarian).

Mix with care and cook only when necessary. Eat only when hungry. Avoid the use of seasonings such as artificial chemicals and salt. Sprinkle liberally with herbs. Which herbs, you may ask?

H for humour many people forget it at the back of the cupboard.

E for enthusiasm we all have but often lose it.

E for exercise we all need but often forget it.

E for encouragement we should all give and receive it.

R for right thinking a positive attitude to problems.

R for relaxation to balance stress.

B for balance the key to health but difficult to achieve all of the time.

S for sociability people need people.

S for supplements to make up for nutrients missing in your diet or to counteract any toxic ones put in.'

Your immune system can be your Achilles' heel or your invincible army. But remember one thing: an army always marches on its stomach. Check that diet!

12
*
THE SECRET SYSTEM

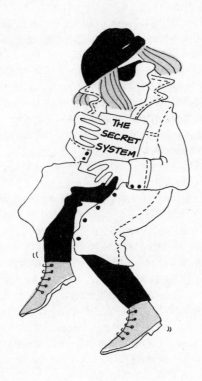

All diseases begin with a loss of energy. It is the universal symptom of something going wrong. Yet how many people feel that they can go to their doctor and complain of a lack of energy? They would prefer to locate their symptoms in one or other area of the body – aching joints, for example, or bad nerves, or a pain in the chest. Initial investigations of these areas often reveal little tangible evidence of illness. Some patients are actually told to go home and come back when they are really ill, while others are given placebos or, worse, a course of tranquillizers or sleeping pills.

When 158 ordinary people were questioned in a survey by the Institute for Optimum Nutrition in London, 92 of them listed lack of energy (sometimes described as tiredness, lack of pep, lassitude) as their overriding symptom. ION and other organizations that deal with contemporary health problems know this to be the norm, and these are so-called healthy people, who are working and walking about.

Observations like this led to the question: is there a system that we are ignoring that is giving us an early warning of what might be avoidable illness? Are we incorrectly attributing symptoms of malaise to other body systems? Could there be a secret controller of them all – an energy system? Energy is, after all, the *modus operandi* of life: the body is a quite simply a factory for making energy. Every day every single cell in your body makes energy. To do this it takes in oxygen (air) in order to burn food (fuel), which gives off heat and energy for life.

For some time now, researchers have been trying to find out how and where that energy flows in the body. They have perceived areas of sickness as being less alive than other areas, paler, with less pulse or somehow stagnant. Commonsense tells them that there is a blockage in the energy flow, yet clearing things like blood vessels, as in heart surgery, does not always improve matters, except in the short term. Similarly, the nervous supply appears to be functioning, yet the block still seems to be there, often manifesting in another place close to the repair.

Gathering evidence piecemeal from all over the globe, scientists began to take interest in evidence coming to light through the practice of alternative medical systems, such as acupuncture, osteopathy and homoeopathy, all of which adhere to one central belief – that in the body there is a life force, the energy of which flows through quite definite channels, closely allied to the circulation and nervous system networks, but not of them.

THE CHINA FACTOR

One of the key factors in this voyage of discovery was occasioned by China opening her doors to the West in the 1970s. Doctors went to

China where they saw patients being treated for a variety of complaints by the simple insertion of a few needles beneath the skin, often in sites of the body quite remote from the source of pain or other symptom! Some patients reported a dramatic remission of symptoms, others improved more slowly, but at no time did the needles enter the organs that were being treated.

They also witnessed major operations conducted without anaesthetic, just with the insertion of a few simple needles containing no drugs, no current and barely penetrating the skin surface! Patients were fully awake, still had movement and feeling, but suffered no pain! Mothers gave birth to babies with full control of their bearing-down muscles during labour – full sensation and consciousness, but no pain.

Medical visitors noticed that post-operative treatment often consisted of 'drugs' that were not strictly drugs, in that they were so dilute that not even one molecule of active chemical could be found in the medicament. Yet case history after case history demonstrated the patient's benefit from the remedy. These were homoeopathic preparations, designed to stimulate the body's own healing resources rather than to control and direct the operation with powerful interventive medicine.

It became clear that actions were being taken which applied themselves to a fundamental force in the body, a force that could heal, a force that could be tapped into in order to block pain signals but without interfering, as would anaesthetics and drugs, with any of the body's processes or sensations. When they were questioned, Chinese doctors produced an age-old map of the body showing a diagram called the acupuncture network, and demonstrated how the deepest of internal organs could be reached and treated by tapping into associated surface points on the skin with tiny needles, in much the same way as one might put a plug into a powerpoint to direct power to an appliance in the home or office!

This network appeared to be just as complex as the blood vessel network or the nervous network, but did not exactly correspond to either of them.

EAST MEETS WEST

Tentatively, doctors began to use acupuncture in the West, at first sceptically, but confidence grew as they saw their patients getting better. This was no miracle treatment, but it certainly was a valuable adjunct to their medical armoury, of especial interest because of the unknown network through which it seemed to operate. It led to questioning and questing that went beyond the therapy to its scientific basis.

As often happens with scientific research, lamps were being lit by investigators in several parts of the world, and one key researcher who was applying himself to yet another aspect of this mysterious energy network, was American orthopaedic surgeon, Dr Robert Becker.

AMERICA ENTERS THE ARENA

Dr Becker was interested in getting the body to mend broken bones better and faster than it sometimes did. In the course of his work with bones, he often came up against the challenging and distressing problem of a patient with a broken bone which refused to knit. In the end the only recourse was amputation.

He began experimenting by implanting tiny wires into the ends of the bones and sending miniscule electric currents through them. To his amazement he was often able to save a patient's limb. Later, he found he was able to speed up healing in patients whose bones knit very slowly. He concluded that somehow he was mimicking a natural healing action of the body that in some patients had flagged.

He turned to old literature on the subject and found that as long ago as the 18th century scientists had discovered that, when the body was injured – skin or bones broken, for example – a tiny current of electricity appeared at the site of the injury and appeared to prompt the healing which took place. If the the current was reversed by external interference healing did not take place.

Becker began to repeat some of the old experiments on salamanders, measuring voltages all along the body, and he discovered the existence of an elaborate field in the form of an organized pattern of electric potentials, which altered in a predictable fashion when the organism was damaged or repairing itself. It also altered when cell division, such as that prior to the production of egg and sperm cells, was taking place.

He noted that this network followed the anatomical arrangement of the nervous system yet appeared to operate independently of it. It seemed as if he had uncovered a 'second nervous system', a data or information system, electrically powered, as is the nervous system, but in this case appearing to regulate activities such as growth and healing through cellular links with the nervous system.

Becker found that tapping into it could change the electric potentials and cut off pain completely. Tapping into it over the brain could send an animal peacefully to sleep to wake up naturally a few hours later.

This discovery of an electronic control system in the body began to throw light on certain mysteries, such as how hypnosis works. As a doctor Becker knew that the states of sleep, anaesthesia and hypnosis all show changes in the electrical potentials in the brain (electroencephalographs reveal this). Similar alterations in consciousness could be brought about, Becker knew, by externally applying appropriate electric currents across the brain. In fact this was a fashionable way of inducing sleep a century or two ago, and may well become so again! These are not strong electric currents but are a bit like ultrasound.

MIND OVER MATTER

In his observations with people, Becker discovered that under hypnosis and in certain altered – calm – states of consciousness such as exist during meditation, these potentials could be altered by an act of the mind. Becker reasoned that since the same electrical system that regulates pain and healing can be demonstrated to come under the control of the mind, it could be a powerful tool for healing and for maintaining the body at high levels of health.

The implications for this in reverse are, of course, that if we consciously or unconsciously implant negative input into a system such as this, then the opposite of health – sickness – could occur. We have arrived by a different track at the beliefs expressed by the new science of psychoneuroimmunology, which demonstrates to us that the mind does indeed influence body states (see Chapters 7 and 11).

This is not to suggest that the mind, through affecting the 'second nervous system' is the sole cause of sickness or health. We have seen how other factors, such as diet, environment, drugs, fitness or rest, etc., have all been shown to play their part. But it does suggest that the mind is a powerful tool in healing.

Becker's work, further substantiated over the past 10 or 20 years by the invention of instruments delicate enough to measure the body's tiny electrical currents (which are so weak they are measured in nano-amperes and microvolts), has formed the foundation of a completely different system of medicine.

THE NEW MEDICINE

Called energy medicine, or vitalistic medicine, it is based on the principle that there is a life force or energy network in the body, that it is susceptible to input from a variety of sources, including stress and pollution, especially electromagnetic pollution such as from VDU or television screens because it itself is electromagnetic in nature, and that in the future any therapy should be directed primarily at keeping this network healthy, because it in turn stimulates and supports all growth, maintenance and healing processes in the body.

I have called this network the secret system because its existence, although long suspected, has remained a secret shared by few.

However, most refer to it as the life force or energy system. A handful of exceptional men such as Reich, Mesmer, Samuel Hahnemann (the father of homoeopathy), de la Warr, Edward Bach (of the Bach flower remedies) and a few others have kept the life-force flame alight through the long dark ages of reductionist medicine, which, of course, denies the existence of a life force and claims that man is simply a collection of organs and that, when they get diseased, the focus of attention should be on the disease, not on the person who has the disease. In other words, man is not greater than the sum of the parts. However we know now that this is not the case.

But let us not crticize a system that has given us such valuable medical assets as penicillin and other powerful antibiotics, which have contributed so much to the control of infectious diseases, or the amazing surgical techniques which can save countless lives that would otherwise be beyond saving. There will always be a place for interventive medicine, but it needs to be complemented with a system which recognizes that there is a central organizing force in the body, the life force or energy network.

As we examine the nature of the energy system, it will be seen that paying attention to this will allow us to do the very things we want to do – that is, to practise preventive health with true complementary medicine.

THE AURA, MEANS TO EARLY DIAGNOSIS

All through this book we have been talking about the importance of symptoms. Now we will show that in order to nip illness in the bud you do not even have to experience the symptoms, you just have to observe the aura, or electrical field, around the body. This is because the aura acts as an early-warning system, showing distortions long before physical symptoms develop. But first, a word about how the aura originates.

THE BODY ELECTRIC
That the body is an electrical system has been known for some time; its biochemical reactions produce feeble ionic currents that yield weak magnetic fields. Think of it as billions and millions of times weaker than domestic electricity. A bit like homoeopathic electricity!

It is a law of physics that the movement of any electrical charge, such as occurs in the cells and, in particular, the nervous system and secret system, creates a magnetic field. This field is not perceptible other than by its effects, except under certain conditions.

Take, for example, the field around a magnet – its magnetic field.

That field is so strong that when iron filings are moved in its vicinity they are sucked up by the magnet's unseen force. This force is an effect of the field.

Likewise, the body has an electromagnetic field, which is commonly called the 'aura', and that field represents the state of play within the object creating the field. When we see a person who is particularly well we often remark that she – it's usually a she – positively glows or is blooming with health. Or we may, if it's a he, say 'he's brimming over with energy'. It's as if somehow we 'know' that good health is synonymous with vitality and luminosity. On the other hand, when we feel a person is really below par, even seriously ill unto death, we sometimes remark 'he or she is drained, or fading rapidly'.

Although most people cannot actually see the aura, there are gifted people, psychics, who can. But now techniques such as Kirlian photography enable the body's magnetic field to be photographed and thus made visible to us all. (VOPs may be familiar with the Kirlian photographs of hands and the emanations from them, as the facility for having one's hands photographed by this technique is often made available in health exhibitions.

There is scientific dispute – and always has been – about what exactly is being shown by the Kirlian image. Some say it is just a picture of surface emanations or

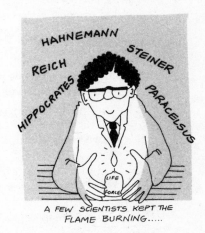

A FEW SCIENTISTS KEPT THE FLAME BURNING.....

corona from an object, but people who have worked with it for years, like British scientist Harry Oldfield, who developed Kirlian photography in the U.K, has seen his Kirlian pictures change to reflect changing states of health in a person under study, and is in no doubt that the technique is giving valuable insight into the internal system. Oldfield points out that just as one's skin reflects one's inner state of health – by its colour, texture, clarity and so on – so do Kirlian pictures of one's outer 'skin', the aura. Anyone wanting to read more about this fascinating subject may like to read my previous book *Life Forces* or Harry's book on his work *The Dark Side of the Brain*.

Leading health expert Jan de Vries, who treats an enormous number of patients weekly at his alternative health clinic in Ayrshire, Scotland, uses Kirlian photography and is very aware of how the extent and strength of the body field can be lowered after a stressful day, even in a healthy person.

In the future, 'aurascopes' could turn out to be as valuable to health as, and a lot less dangerous than, X-rays in that they may be used as a diagnostic tool to check on areas that might give trouble in the future. Treatment can then be arranged to adjust the trouble spot either with acupuncture or with some of the new vibrational therapies that are coming into being.

Will the treatment modes of the future eliminate our necessity ever to feel symptoms? Is it true that mapping auras (or to put it more accurately, the body energy field) will enable us to predict future health problems? In the meantime, it may pay us all to take more notice of our energy-levels than we are wont to do.

UNDERSTANDING YOUR ENERGY

Have you noticed a consistent pattern in your energy levels during the day? Are you a person who needs a boost early in the morning, or are you five o'clock flagger?

The first thing to do is map your own energy pattern. Having done that, observe what you do to give yourself the boost you need when you feel energy flagging.

Does your technique involve any of the following: chocolate, coffee, strong tea, cigarettes, cola, cakes, biscuits, sweets, fizzy drinks or alcohol?

Then you had better know straight away that all these substances are robbers of energy. Their action releases certain powerful hormones into the blood, which will certainly give you a boost, just as, in a more serious way, a shot in the arm gives a drug addict a boost. But the end result is that all this activity drains the body's existing energy supplies but does not facilitate the making of energy. In fact it does the reverse.

This is a bit like living on an overdraft. Every time your bank account gets topped up by your salary cheque above the level agreed by your bank manager, you can draw out a bit more cash, but you never get clear of the debilitating effects of the overdraft or of the charges you are paying for this facility.

What you need is something that increases your basic supply of energy, so that you have a balance of energy in your bank from which to draw. The same principle works for your body.

There are several ways of putting energy on deposit. One sure way is to see that a large part of your diet, up to three-quarters of it, consists of complex carbohydrates, such as vegetables, beans, lentils and whole grains such as brown rice. These the body views as ideal 'fuel' for its energy-producing activities, since they are 'slow-burners', releasing energy-producing glucose into the bloodstream in a consistent manner. Whereas foods or stimulants such as those mentioned above cause energy to be released into the bloodstream in too rapid a manner, with the result that the body over-reacts and releases hormones, which not only reduce the glucose level but do so excessively, creating a slump in energy between one to three hours after eating. This results in more craving for the very things that are causing this effect. It is especially true of sugar and sugary products.

KICKING THE SUGAR HABIT

Kicking the sugar habit, like kicking any habit, is not easy, and to a certain extent you have got to ease yourself out of it. Do not, whatever you do, use sugar substitutes (except in the very early stages); not only are these bad for you, but in substituting another sweetness they fail to re-educate your palate, so that you stay a sweet-tooth and therefore always vulnerable.

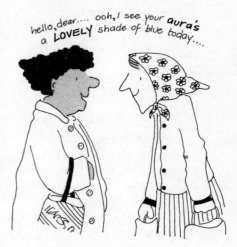

Get a supply of sun-dried, not sulphur-dried, fruit such as Hunza apricots and use these. Take two raisins in your mouth or three of four sultanas. Do limit yourself! Suck a piece of dried apple, have a few hazelnuts or almonds (these are sweetish). As your sugar craving slowly diminishes, you will find that you get to the point where you cannot imagine how you liked the sweet things you once lived on.

SECOND LINE ENERGY ROBBERS

Although coffee, cocoa, tea, cola and even diabetic chocolate may not contain sugar as such, they cause exactly the same reaction because they are stimulants. Through the same 'emergency' channels (see Chapter 7 and stress) they stimulate the liver and other tissues to release glucose rapidly into the bloodstream. The result is that the bloodstream gets flooded again, over controlled again, and we are left with an energy slump shortly afterwards. Furthermore, these substances are doubly draining because they are empty of minerals and vitamins, requiring the body to use up its own supplies to make energy.

The above situation also applies to nicotine (see Chapter 6) and some commonly used remedies such as aspirin.

THE OXYGEN FACTOR

In order to burn food to make energy, the body needs the vital ingredient of oxygen. Since we breathe in a fairly consistent manner, it might be considered that oxygen is supplied on a steady basis, but the problem here is one of quantity. If we are slumped over in a chair, breathing shallowly, minimal oxygen is available to the cells. This is why we feel so much better when in the open air; the freshness encourages us to breathe more deeply and the result is more energy. So remember to take a few, good, deep breaths every so often to increase energy supplies.

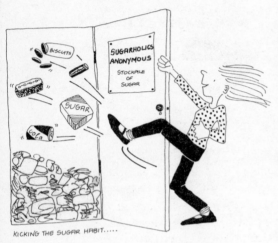

KICKING THE SUGAR HABIT.....

THE EXERCISE EQUATION

A third factor is exercise, which stimulates the system to release energy. Ten minutes' work-out will get you going in the morning and can, if not taken too late, promote healthy sleep at night.

The best exercise is that which makes you breathe deeply and increases your stamina, such as brisk walking, swimming, trampolining, skipping, cycling and jogging (with some reservations; see Chapter 8). If you cannot face this (ask yourself why!) try at least to walk up a flight of stairs where you would normally have taken the elevator. Walk briskly to work. Go for a walk at lunch time. Talk yourself into doing something.

ENERGY-DRAINING FOOD ALLERGIES AND HOW TO IDENTIFY THEM

Food allergies are becoming more and more frequent as scientists and food growers and producers tamper with raw materials such as grains. There are two simple ways in which you can find out which foods may be draining you and which are all right, apart, that is, from observing your own energy reaction after eating them. The first is applied kinesiology or muscle testing. For this you require the cooperation of an expert, but you will not have to go back and back. The technique is unbelivably simple – so simple, in fact, that it is hard to believe it works. Believe me, it does.

While you go through a list of foods you eat, the muscle tester stands beside you and tests your muscular strength as each food is mentioned. The technique for doing this varies slightly, but it usually involves the deltoid muscle in the upper arm. This muscle seems to have a special link with the unconscious, and when a food is mentioned that the unconscious knows to be bad, the muscles reveal the stress by weakening momentarily when gentle pressure is applied to it by the tester.

Alternatively, you may have a dowser dowse the foods you eat through linking in to you by a hair sample. Some foods on the black list will not surprise you in the least; others will raise your eyebrows as you either like them or appear to eat them without reaction. In the case of some deep-seated allergies, the body has simply given up reacting against them, rather as you might decide not to argue with certain people because it is a waste of time! Nevertheless, these aggravating factors affect the system and its energy.

ILLNESS: THE ULTIMATE ENERGY-DRAINER

It is surprising how few people realize that fighting illness drains energy. They seem to associate the illness itself with the lack of energy rather than the fact that it is the struggle that uses up the body's reserves. A tremendous number of cells have to be made in order to top up the ranks of the immune system, and, toxins have to be eliminated. All of this takes energy, which is why we should rest when we are ill, not carry on.

THE MIND AND ENERGY; THE REAL BRAIN-DRAIN

Never underestimate the power of the mind over the body. Getting caught up in a vortex of negative thoughts and negative patterns of action can, literally, drain your energy bank. Most people can remember just how ill and drained they have felt after a terrible argument. This is a big energy drain and as such we notice it; but what about the countless little ones that occur daily? We cannot avoid them, but we can stop letting them drag us down.

The whole purpose of this book has been to encourage self-help and self understanding. Now is a good time to write your own list of energy-destroying habits. Why not do this exercise with your family?

Make a list of what you feel to be your own energy-draining habits.

Leave space at the bottom of the list for your family to fill in their opinions. All of you do likewise – or do so anonymously if you prefer! In any case, agree not to argue if you show your lists to each other – you are trying to help, not obstruct each other. You may decide to name and pool the lists and look at them in your own quiet moments. This way you achieve family feed-back and initial privacy while you absorb what others have had to say!

After due consideration, you may want to re-do your list. You may not agree with something your family has on it. Put the final version in a place that you frequent. When you are particularly upset, try to remember that list and see if you're not making matters worse by an attitude you would like to change.

I made such a list as a young woman in a moment of absolute clear perception. I smile sometimes at how close to the mark I was! Fortunately, you never quite forget such an exercise – something of it lingers to remind you not to be quite so wasteful of energy in future.

THE FOUR FUNDAMENTS OF PRESERVING YOUR LIFE FORCE

Jung said we had four ways of expressing ourselves in life, four ways in which we function – thinking, feeling, sensing (i.e. sensation), and intuiting.

We need to express all four functions if our lifestyle is to be balanced. We need to support our sensation function by eating, touching and making love. We need to stretch our minds and use our thinking function. We need to feel, to care for someone and to be cared for. And we need a spiritual component in our lives, a belief in the intangible, which is what modern life most lacks. However, our intuition continues to teach us, by showing us that our hunches are often right and that there are more things than we can perceive with our other senses. The function you feel is most lacking in your life is probably the one from which you will derive most help in the therapeutic sense. So, if you feel that your life lacks a spiritual component, you may find that spiritual healing is of tremendous help to you, or a spiritual pursuit, even if it is only visiting mediums or reading books on psychics or learning astrology!

If you feel you are not getting enough sensation of the touching kind in your life, seek a touch therapy such as reflexology (read more about that in Chapter 8) or choose aromatherapy or massage.

If you have difficulty in expressing your feelings, which many men do, consider listening to music, having psychotherapy (it may save you from surgery later) or simply trying to say how you feel. Sometimes practice is all that is needed.

If you feel your brain is stultifying (this happens to women bringing up a young family), join a study group in the evenings or try to read one book a week on a subject that fascinates you. Take up a hobby, learn by correspondence.

These may seem funny ways to generate energy – by expending it – but we all know how much better we feel when something has stimulated us to actually **do** something about our torpor.

Finally, try to cut out the chemical props in your life because they are almost certainly polluting your inner sea as surely as they are polluting the seas of the world. Remember, some of the biggest energy drainers of all are tranquillizers and sleeping pills, so try to give them up. Caution! Do not do this alone; seek medical sanction or approach one of the organizations listed in Useful Addresses.

Remember that at the intervention stage, which is the basis for prescribing of most allopathic medicines, drugs have to be so powerful that they literally pow you. Build up your energy and it will empower you to solve your own personal energy crisis.

13
*
THERE MUST BE MORE TO HEALTH THAN WEALTH

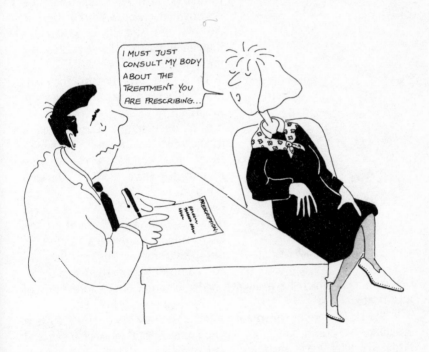

Now that you have read the salient parts of this book, you are going to have to decide how – if at all – you plan to change your habits and lifestyle.

You will also have to decide whom you will have to support you in this venture – what therapists, what type of medical advice, what insurance and so on. It is quite a complex matter. Being part of a changing pattern of healthcare, whether you decide to opt in now or later – or, like Colossus, try to keep astride of both systems – will involve you in more decision-making than you have ever had to consider before about health.

But one thing is certain: as we approach the 21st century, we do so in the sure knowledge that the existing medical/health system will have

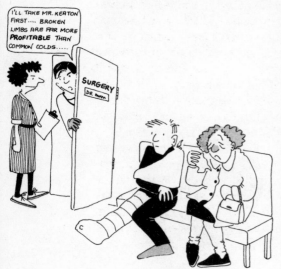

to change in order to incorporate a system that embraces both preventive medicine and the understanding that 'each patient is to be treated, not the disease'.

These are two massive molehills from which to try and move the mountain of existing orthodox practice of interventive, disease-centred medicine. Speaking both on a personal and general level, we are bound to have to go through troubled times in order to get the health care we both need and deserve. For European countries, the EEC further complicates matters as our health representatives strive to find common ground between member countries which have always had their individual expressions of healthcare.

In the UK, where the alternative tradition has always been strong and available, we are in danger of having some of our most effective and distinctive alternative treatments and remedies cut out by the newly developing establishment that is controlling the EEC's health policies. This is in addition to our battle with the existing medical establishment within the UK, as it strives to maintain the *status quo* against the progress dictated by a new understanding of health. The current debate about the closing of some of London's longest established hospitals, which cost a fortune to run and can treat only a tiny minority of the general public, is a classic example of the existing dilemma between keeping the best of the old, established, interventive medicine while making room for the new, preventive medicine and healthcare.

In the USA, the battle with the establishment will have to be fought on the commercial level, against the vastly powerful drug companies that control many medical decisions. It may also have to be fought against the makers of medical equipment, which in the future will be simpler and much less costly – scanning devices, for example, are likely to cost a fraction of what they have done.

Commonwealth countries and the rest of the Western world will all have their own problems to sort out, but it would be true to say that at the moment most healthcare systems are run on a purely commercial basis, and this is no longer good enough where health is concerned – there must be more to health than wealth.

However, in countries where this principle has been recognized, such as in Britain, which has a National Health Service, the real has fallen short of the ideal, probably because the National Health was based on a system which did not address modern problems (see Chapter 1). This is now being realized and definite steps are being taken to introduce preventive health measures into the existing system, and to change it in other ways to provide much-needed community care.

But where does this leave the individual? Helpless – to be carried along on the ebb and flow of the changes, recessions and upheavals that will inevitably take place before the new systems are instated?

Hopefully not, but the role of the individual may have to be very much more active than before. People will have to become more self-preservationist. Fortunately this works well with what we now know about health – that it is up to the individual to maintain healthy habits of diet, lifestyle, anti-pollution home and personal measures in order to stay healthy. If we follow regimes such as those suggested in this book we may rarely need to become patients in a doctor's surgery.

SELF-HELP HEALTH

Why this book has been written about self-help and self-sufficiency in health matters must now be obvious. Hopefully it has also whetted your appetite to learn more about your body, since it is indeed a fascinating study.

In fact, I believe that physiology, the study of the body, plus what keeps it healthy, should be taught in schools as a compulsory subject, and that the experience of the team that has brought the Life Education programmes to schools to try to combat the terrifying drug threat to our next generation is showing us just the way to do it – that is, to use a knowledge of the body and its miraculous workings to promote both respect and careful maintenance of it.

With time and knowledge on our side, we can use medical and other health professionals as we use lawyers or financial consultants, to get advice, consider, then decide what health measures we wish to take. Preventive healthcare gives us that time, because we do not have to wait until we are really sick before getting help, by which time we may be disempowered and desperate.

But what of those tied to an insurance scheme structured to treat under the techniques of conventional medicine? Or those served by a government health scheme such as the National Health Service in Britain? The first thing anyone who is tied to conventional healthcare can do is to find out what is available on it. Alternative treatment modes, such as acupuncture, personal counselling, massage and relaxation training, are increasingly accessible. Homoeopathy is an alternative form of medicine that is available within the conventional system. In the UK such treatment lies within National Health options.

Find out which of these options your health system offers – you may be pleasantly surprised. In the UK a booklet is available from the Health Service; it is entitled *The NHS Reforms and You* and is published by the Central Office of Information and available at council and community centres. No doubt there are similar publications describing health advancements in every Commonwealth country and in America.

The UK booklet concentrates on the new prevention aspect of health and details services that promote this cause, such as smear tests and breast screening for women, family planning, immunization, heart health checks, dietary guides and child health care. Many people are unaware of just how much help is available to them if only they would ask at their local community care centre or council.

Another booklet, the Patients' Charter, which is similarly available, should be in the possession of every household. This tells you your rights as a patient and what options are available to you, should you receive treatment which you deem to be unsatisfactory.

Very often, the problem with people who have reached the stage of ill-health where they require treatment, perhaps hospitalization, is that they no longer have the stamina to enforce their right of choice. This is why it is so important to take a strong and healthy ally with you when you are going for a key consultation about your health, and before you go to list the questions you wish to have answered.

ABOUT DOCTORS

There is a good deal of criticism about doctors these days, and much of it stems from displeasure with a system they represent rather than with their individual contribution.

Doctors are human (sometimes superhuman). They are busy people trying to do their best, often with insufficient information, both about you and about the medication/treatment they are considering for you. They do not know your body, they only know the average human body. You are individual in more ways than your personality. The sum total of everything you have ever thought, eaten and experienced is reflected in your body, and only you know how it feels under certain circumstances.

Because of this your help and cooperation may be needed in order to arrive at the best possible decision about how to treat your problem. So do not sit there mute; tell the doctor how you feel, and say if any treatment or medication has disagreed with you in the past.

Though it may be hard to stand up to your doctor and question him or her when you are sick and need help, do understand that it may be just as hard for your doctor to show sympathy when all he or she sees are sick people, day in, day out! So make your requests brief and without prejudice – you will probably get an unprejudiced response.

The minute you leave the surgery with your diagnosis and your prescription, don't let it rest there. Start reading about your complaint. If you were too shy to ask the doctor, ask the chemist about the tablets you have been given. Ask at your pharmacy or your local health shop if there are alternative herbal preparations for your complaint. If your tablets don't suit you, or when you have finished them, you may like to try the alternative. But first you should have established with your doctor how important, in his or her opinion, your medication is.

PERSUASION v. INVASION

It is important to realize when you are trying alternative remedies to allopathic drugs that we have all got used to allopathic medicine and we expect to feel something – even if it is only worse! Allopathic drugs are strong. They don't coax the body; instead, by and large they push (and bush) it. It will take a while to re-condition your body (and yourself) not to feel something when you take a herbal or homoeopathic medicine. At first they may seem to do no good: they take time, because they let your body make the pace.

BODY LANGUAGE
Start talking to your body; start thinking of it as a person – an identity. People have done so with other 'pet' pieces of machinery such as their cars – which is very interesting, because it is a mark of respect, of affection – making some of us wonder, surely, whether we have ever respected that Rolls Royce of equipment, our body.

When considering a treatment or action, ask the body how it feels about it in a quiet moment. It will answer you; you may not like the answer, but you will get one! A trick to testing whether a food, drink or action is good for you is to first ask yourself if you like it and second ask is it really good for me? The answer to the second question is likely to be the body replying!

TREATMENT OPTIONS

Deciding on a diet, a course of action, the treatment, an exercise programme and so on to improve and maintain your health is a complex matter, one in which trial and error will have to play a part. With luck you will get advice from many quarters, and you will hear many stories along the road that bear witness to the success of one or other treatment diets or remedies. There are people who were at death's door who have been cured by the Hay diet (food combining) and equally there are people who have been at death's door who have been cured by almost every other kind of diet, or no diet at all . . . the point is that there are many roads to the Rome of good health: yours is your individual route.

Never be afraid to try something (or someone) new. In fact, if your doctor loses interest in you, it is probably wise to move on. It is an unfortunate patient who frustrates his doctors by not getting well as quickly as they would like.

As you begin to get better, you may be surprised and taken aback by getting old symptoms and sometimes quite acute mini-illnesses back again. In order to cure itself once and for all the body has to go through a repeat performance in which it wins the battle it could not win before. Mostly these recur in reverse order of getting them, but sometimes the body skips a sequence, either because it cannot address it in order or because it has not got the necessary spare parts to effect a repair.

PRESENCE OF THE PAST

Not everything will be completely cured unless you are very young, very assiduous with your health routines or very lucky. The presence of the past is always with us reminding us of our progress in life.

As I sit writing this last chapter and I mentally take stock of my own body, which has been groaning because of too much word-processing, I can still feel residues from some of the health conditions from which I have suffered in the past. Of others, not. And I can honestly say that ALL of my still-existing health conditions have been caused by wrong treatment, usually too harsh.

Do I blame the professionals who used my body to such disadvantage? No. I blame myself, for putting my body into their hands without trying to learn anything about my complaint. Blindly or blandly I took myself to their consulting rooms and became an accomplice in what they did. The law has always known that ignorance is no defence. Now we, the ordinary people, must know it about our health.

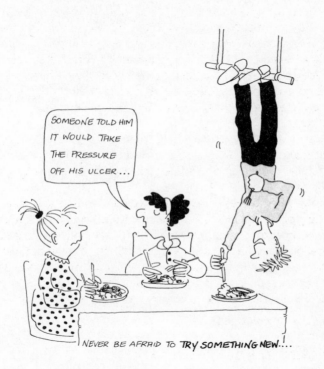

USEFUL ADDRESSES

Do be sure to enclose a stamped, self-addressed envelope with your enquiry; most of these organizations work on a shoe-string.

Nutritional Suppliers
General vitamins and minerals

Nature's Best Health Products Ltd
1 Lambert's Road
PO Box 1
Tunbridge Wells TN2 3EQ
(Nutritional advisor available)

General supplies, including lecithin

Solgar Vitamins (UK) Ltd
Solgar House
Chiltern Commerce Centre
Asheridge Road
Chesham
Bucks HP5 2PY
(Also found in most health stores
and some large chemists, including
John, Bell & Croyden, 50 Wigmore
Street, London W1H 0AU)

*Enzymes, acidophilus and
digestive aids,
hypoallergenic/children's vitamins
and minerals*

Bio Care
54 Northfield Road
King's Norton
Birmingham B30 1JH

**Suppliers of Herbs and
Adaptogen Products**

Brazilian herbs

Rio Trading Company (Health) Ltd
Rio House
2 Eaton Place
Brighton
East Sussex BN2 1EH

*Specialist herb tinctures such as
Echinaforce, Symphosan (for
arthritis), Shark Liver Oil, Green
Lipped Mussel*

Bioforce (UK) Ltd
Olympic Business Park
Dundonald
Ayrshire KA2 9BE

Natural medicines and toiletries

Weleda (UK) Ltd
Heanor Road
Ilkeston
Derbyshire DE7 8DR

*Royal jelly, ginseng, pollen and
other bee products*

Ortis
P.O. Box 223A
Thames Ditton
Surrey KT7 0LY

Suppliers of Equipment

Full-spectrum light

True-lite

	Unit 1, Riverside Business Centre Victoria Street High Wycombe Bucks HP11 2LT
	Wholistic Research Company (see below)
Water purifiers	General Ecology Unit 8, Orwell Close Fairview Industrial Park Manor Way Rainham Essex RN13 8UB
Water distillers, air purifiers and juicers	Wholistic Research Co. Bright Haven Robin's Lane Lolworth Cambridge CB3 8HH
Biofeedback devices and information	Biomonitors 26 Wendell Road London W12 9RT
Electro-crystal Therapy and Kirlian Treatment Devices	School of Electro-crystal Therapy 117 Long Drive South Ruislip HA4 0HL
Skin brushing and colonic cleansing herbs	G & G Food Supplies Ltd 175 London Road East Grinstead West Sussex RH19 1YY

Treatment Centres and Services

Complementary Medicine	Centre for the Study of Complementary Medicine 51 Bedford Place Southampton SO1 2DG (Medical practitioners using bio-regulatory and diagnostic equipment such as Vega; also homoeopathy) also at:
	14 Harley House Upper Harley Street off Marylebone Road London NW1 4PR
	Marylebone Health Centre and Trust 17 Marylebone Road London NW1 5LT
Homoeopathy	Register of Professionals Society of Homoeopaths 2 Artizan Road Northampton NN1 4HU

221

	For treatment contact nearest homoeopathic hospital; in the UK in London, Glasgow, Liverpool, Bristol and Tunbridge Wells. Or write to: British Homoeopathic Association 27A Devonshire Street London W1N 1RJ
General alternative therapies	Hale Clinic 7 Park Crescent London W1N 3HE
Anthroposophical medicine (based on Rudolf Steiner's approach)	Park Attwood Clinic Trimpley Bewdley Worcestershire DY12 1RE
	Rudolf Steiner House Anthroposophical Society in Great Britain 35 Park Road London NW1 6XT
Alternative therapy clinic	Jan de Vries Auchenkyle Southwoods Road Troon Ayrshire KA10 7EL
Herbal therapy	National Institute of Medical Herbalists Ltd 9 Palace Gate Exeter Devon EX1 1JA
Nutrition (general)	Institute for Optimum Nutrition 5 Jerdan Place London SW6 1BE (Hair analysis undertaken)
Allergies	Dr Jean Munro Breakspear Hospital High Street Abbotts Langley Herts WD5 0PU
Gerson Cancer Therapy	The Gerson Institute P.O. Box 430 Bonita CA 02002 USA (Book available from P. A. Faulkner, 57 Bridge St, Pershore, Worcs. WR10 1AL)

Alternative treatments for cancer, AIDS etc	Naessens c/o Weikang Ltd 7 Elderpark Workspace 100 Elderpark Street Glasgow G51 3TR
Hormone replacement therapy	Amarant Trust 56-60 St John St London EC1M 4DT
	Marie Stopes Clinic 108 Whitfield Street London W1P 6BE (General health care for women. Also in Leeds and Manchester.)
Osteoporosis: prevention, detection and treatment	The Endocrine Centre 69 Wimpole Street London W1M 7DE
PMT (nutritional advice)	Women's Nutritional Advisory Service PO Box 268 Lewes BN7 2QN
Chelation	Marie Stopes Clinics (see above)
	Arterial Diseases Clinic 3rd Floor, 57A Wimpole Street London W1M 7DF
	70 The Avenue Leigh Lancashire WN7 1ET
	Arterial Health Foundation PO Box 8 Atherton Manchester M29 9FY
Colonic irrigation	Colonics International Hydrotherapy Foundation 57A Warwick Avenue London W9 2PS
	Hale Clinic (see above) (both use disposables and hydrotherapy machines)
	Colonics International Association 50A Morrish Road London SW2 4EG
Stop smoking	Full Stop PO Box 2484 London N6 5UX

223

Psychotherapy/counselling	The Westminster Pastoral Foundation 23 Kensington Square London W8 5HN
	British Association for Counselling 1 Regent Place Rugby Warwickshire CV21 2PJ
Breathing/hyperventilation tapes	British Holistic Medical Association 179 Gloucester Place London NW1 6DX
Anti-drug mobile education for children	Life Education Centres PO Box 137 London N10 3JJ
Dentists who are aware of amalgam toxicity	British Dental Society for Clinical Nutrition Flat 1, Welbeck House 62 Welbeck Street London W1M 7HB
Tranquillizer addiction	Council for Involuntary Tranquillizer Addiction Cavendish House Brighton Road Waterloo Liverpool L22 5NG
	Natural Medicines Society Edith Lewis House Back Lane Ilkeston Derbyshire DE7 8EJ (For booklet on alternative approaches to addiction; sae please)
	MIND (National Association for Mental Health) 22 Harley Street London W1N 2ED (Will give local branches or therapist)
Transcendental Meditation	Transcendental Meditation Network Freepost London SW1P 4YY (for information pack and details of your local centre)

Groups and Associations

Kinesiology	Association for Systematic Kinesiology 39 Brown's Road

Surbiton
Surrey KT5 8ST

Dowsing

British Society of Dowsers
Sycamore Barn
Tamley Lane
Hastingleigh
Ashford
Kent TN25 5HW

Aromatherapy

International Federation of
    Aromatherapists
Room 8
Department of Continuing Education
Royal Masonic Hospital
Ravenscourt Park
London W6 OTN

Register of Qualified Aromatherapists
52 Barrack Lane
Aldwick
Bognor Regis
West Sussex PO21 4DD

Reflexology

Association of Reflexologists
27 Old Gloucester Street
London WC1N 3XX

British Reflexology Association
Monks Orchard
Whitbourne
Worcestershire WR6 5RB

Alexander Technique

The Society of Teachers of the
    Alexander Technique
20 London House
266 Fulham Road
London SW10 9EL

Candida

The Hale Clinic (see above) and
most local naturopathic clinics can
treat candida.

ME

ME Association
Stanhope House
High Street
Stanford le Hope
Essex SS17 0HA

Seasonal Affective Disorder

SAD Association
P.O. Box 989
London SW7 2P2

Acupuncture (there are several
associations, of which this is one)

British Acupuncture Association
34 Alderney Street
London SW1V 4EU
(For list of practitioners send £2.30)

Physiotherapists	Chartered Society of Physiotherapists 14 Bedford Row London WC1R 4ED
Osteopathy	Osteopathic Information Service 37 Soho Square London W1V 5DG.
Cranial osteopaths	Cranial Osteopathic Association 478 Baker Street Enfield Middlesex EN1 3QS
Chiropractors	British Chiropractic Association 29 Whitley Street Reading RG2 0EG
	Institute of Pure Chiropractic 14 Park End Street Oxford OX1 1HH

FURTHER READING

Where possible the cheapest or most up-to-date edition has been given rather than the first edition. Some titles listed are currently out of print, but most will be available from good libraries.

Brown, Richard, *Conquering Heart and Artery Disease*, Arterial Health Foundation, Atherton, 1990.

Cannon, Geoffrey and Enzig, Hetty, *Dieting Makes You Fat*, Sphere, London, 1984.

Collings, Jillie, *Life Forces*, New English Library, London, 1991

Cooper, Wendy, *No Change: Biological Revolution for Women*, revised edn, Arrow Books, London, 1983.

Diamond, Harvey and Marilyn, *Fit for Life*, Bantam, London, 1987

Gerson, Max, *Cancer Therapy: Results of Fifty Cases*, available from P. A. Faulkner, 57 Bridge St, Pershore, Worcs. WR10 1AL

Gillett, Richard, *Overcoming Depression*, British Holistic Medical Association in association with Dorling Kindersley Ltd, London, 1987

Grant, Doris, and Joice, Jean *Food Combining for Health*, Thorsons Publishers Ltd, Wellingborough, 1984

Hanson, Peter, *The Joy of Stress*, Pan Books Ltd, London, 1987

Hauser, Gayelord, *Look Younger, Live Longer*, Faber & Faber, London, 1973

Hay, Louise, *You Can Heal Your Life*, Eden Grove Editions, London, 1988 (first published in the U.S.A. by Hay House Inc.)

Holford, Patrick, *Supernutrition for a Healthy Heart*, ION Press, London, 1989

Keay, Sarah, *Back in Action*, Century, London, 1991

Kilmartin, Angela, *Understanding Cystitis*, revised edn, Arrow Books, London 1989 (first published by Heinemann, London, 1973)

Kowalski, Robert E., *The 8 Week Cholesterol Cure*, Thorsons Publishers Ltd, Wellingborough, 1988

Leboyer, Frederick, *Birth Without Violence*, Fontana, London, 1977 (first published in France under the title *Pour une Naissance sans Violence*, Editions de Seuil, Paris, 1974)

Martlew, Gillian, and Silver, Shelley, *The Pill Protection Plan*, Grapevine (Thorsons Publishers Ltd). Wellingborough, 1989

Meek, Jennifer, *How to Boost Your Immune System*, ION Press, London, 1988

Munro, Jean, and Mansfield, Peter, *Chemical Children*, Century Hutchinson, London, 1987

Odent, Michel, *Birth Reborn*, Fontana, London, 1986

Oldfield, Harry, and Coghill, Roger, *The Dark Side of the Brain*, Element Books, Shaftesbury, Dorset, 1988

Riley, Gillian, *How to Stop Smoking and Stay Stopped for Good*, Vermilion, London, 1992

Roberts, Gwylim, *Boost Your Child's Brain Power*, Thorsons Publishers Ltd, Wellingborough, 1988

Trickett, Shirley, *Coming off Tranquillizers and Sleeping Pills*, Thorsons Publishers Ltd, Wellingborough, 1986

Vries, Jan de, *Neck and Back Problems*, Mainstream Publishing Co., Edinburgh, 1987

Young, Jacqueline, *Self-Massage*, Thorsons Publishers Ltd, London, 1992

Yudkin, John, *Pure, White and Deadly*, Penguin Books, Harmondsworth, 1988

INDEX